DIAGNOSTIC

ENDOCRINOLOGY

D.C. Evered
BSc, MD, FRCP, FIBiol
Second Secretary,
Medical Research Council

R. Hall
CBE, BSc, MD, FRCP
Emeritus Professor of Medicine,
University of Wales College of Medicine

Wolfe Publishing Ltd

Titles in this series, published or being developed, include:
Picture Tests in Human Anatomy
Diagnostic Picture Tests in Oral Medicine
Diagnostic Picture Tests in Orthopaedics
Diagnostic Picture Tests in Infectious Diseases
Diagnostic Picture Tests in Dermatology
Diagnostic Picture Tests in Ophthalmology
Diagnostic Picture Tests in Rheumatology
Diagnostic Picture Tests in Obstetrics/Gynaecology
Diagnostic Picture Tests in Clinical Neurology
Diagnostic Picture Tests in Injury in Sport
Diagnostic Picture Tests in General Surgery
Diagnostic Picture Tests in General Medicine
Diagnostic Picture Tests in Paediatric Dentistry
Diagnostic Picture Tests in Paediatrics
Diagnostic Picture Tests in Ear, Nose & Throat
Diagnostic Picture Tests in Urology

Copyright © 1991 Wolfe Publishing Ltd
Published by Wolfe Publishing Ltd, 1991
Printed by BPCC Hazell Books, Aylesbury, England
ISBN 0 7234 1701 6

A CIP catalogue record for this book is available from the British Library.

For a full list of Atlases in the series, plus forthcoming titles and details of
our surgical, dental and veterinary Atlases, please write to
Wolfe Publishing Ltd, Brook House, 2–16 Torrington Place,
London WC1E 7LT, England.

Preface

Diagnostic Picture Tests in Endocrinology is meant to complement *A Colour Atlas of Endocrinology,* Second Edition, by R. Hall and D. Evered. We have adopted a problem-solving approach using a variety of multiple-choice question formats. We hope that this will provide a relaxed, informative method of revision for medical students and for postgraduates studying for higher examinations. We have tried to deal largely with common endocrine problems and have generally avoided the more abstruse byways of endocrinology. Nonetheless the questions cover a range of difficulty from the routine clinical to the scholarship level. Most of the questions test clinical diagnostic ability and also background knowledge of the conditions and approaches to laboratory diagnosis and treatment. The answers give details of the modern background to the clinical management of endocrine disease.

D.C. Evered, London
R. Hall, Cardiff

Acknowledgements

We are pleased to acknowledge the provision of slides by our many colleagues listed in the second edition of *A Colour Atlas of Endocrinology* and the help and cooperation of Professor Ralph Marshall and the Department of Medical Illustration at the University of Wales College of Medicine.

1

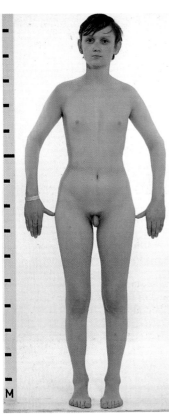

1 This 22-year-old man complained of lack of sexual development. He was of normal height, but clearly hypogonadal with a small penis and testes, each 2 ml in volume and soft. Which of the following statements about his assessment are true?

(i) Enquiry should be made as to episodes of pain and swelling of the testes and of mumps orchitis.

(ii) He should be asked about his sense of smell.

(iii) His other pituitary functions should be assessed clinically.

(iv) He is likely to be suffering from panhypopituitarism.

(v) Measurement of plasma testosterone, serum luteinizing hormone and follicle-stimulating hormone would be helpful.

2

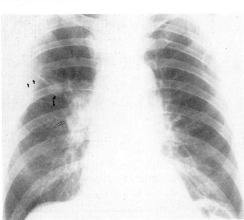

2 (a) What is this chest lesion?

(b) Which of the following endocrine disorders may be associated with this chest lesion: diabetes mellitus, Conn's syndrome, Cushing's syndrome, hyperglycaemia, Addison's disease?

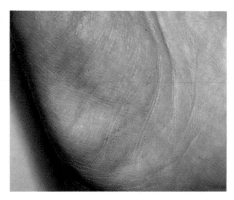

3 (a) What physical sign is illustrated in this hand and to what is it usually due?

(b) Which of the following statements about this condition are true?

(i) An underlying cause can almost always be recognised.

(ii) It is commonly seen in acromegaly.

(iii) Surgical treatment is almost always required.

(iv) Nerve conduction studies are no help in establishing the diagnosis.

(v) The symptoms tend to be worse in bed at night.

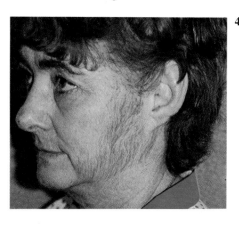

4 (a) What clinical abnormality is illustrated in this picture?

(b) Which of the following drugs are known to cause this condition: diazoxide, phenytoin, paracetamol, prednisolone, cyclosporin A?

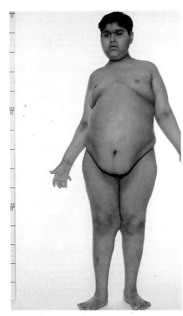

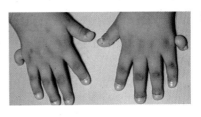

5, 6 This adolescent boy presented with hypopituitarism and mental retardation.
(a) What is the clinical diagnosis?
(b) What are the clinical features illustrated in these pictures and what is the site of the lesion?

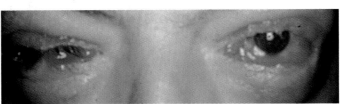

7 (a) This 35-year-old woman, a known case of Graves' disease, had been treated with an ablative dose of radioiodine for hyperthyroidism 6 months previously. For 2 months she had complained of progressive swelling, watering and pain in the eyes and for one week had been unable to read. She was clinically and biochemically mildly hyperthyroid. What is the diagnosis?
(b) Which of the following statements about this condition are correct?
    (i) It is a medical emergency requiring immediate admission to a specialised endocrine unit.
    (ii) There is no risk to vision as the condition will remit with thyroxine medication.
    (iii) Papilloedema is invariably present.
    (iv) Macular oedema plays no part in the visual failure.
    (v) Defects in colour vision may be present.

8 This man presented with temporal headaches. He had a sister who had had an operation on her neck for reasons unknown, and who had passed multiple stones in her urine.

(a) What are the likely diagnoses in the man and his sister and what condition must be considered?

(b) Which of the following disorders are associated with this condition:

  (i) prolactinomas,

  (ii) Cushing's disease,

  (iii) hyperparathyroidism,

  (iv) medullary carcinoma of the thyroid,

  (v) islet-cell tumours of the pancreas,

  (vi) adrenocortical adenomas?

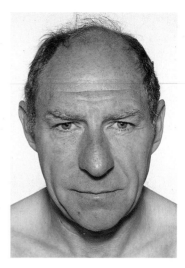

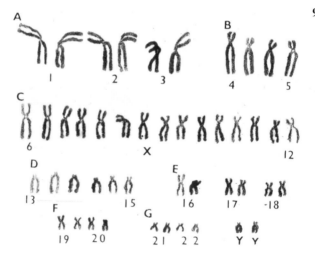

9 The karyotype shown is XYY. Which of the following characteristics may be associated with this abnormality:

  (i) aggressive behaviour,

  (ii) schizophrenia,

  (iii) shortness of stature,

  (iv) capillary haemangiomata,

  (v) varicosities of the superficial veins?

10

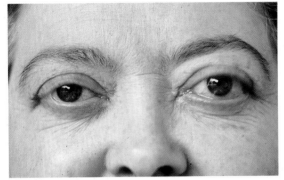

11

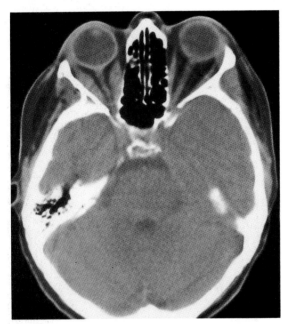

10, 11 (a) A 40-year-old woman's only complaint was
of swelling of the left eye of 3 months' duration (**10**).
She was clinically and biochemically euthyroid, but
her serum showed a high titre of thyroid peroxidase
antibodies. What is the likely diagnosis?
(b) What does her CT scan (**11**) show and does it help
to confirm the diagnosis?

12 (a) What is the probable diagnosis in this man who has been receiving no medication?
(b) Which of the following investigations are essential to confirm or refute the diagnosis:
  (i) serum sodium concentration,
  (ii) plasma ACTH concentration,
  (iii) morning plasma cortisol concentration,
  (iv) 24-hour urinary free cortisol concentration,
  (v) measurement of circadian rhythm of cortisol?

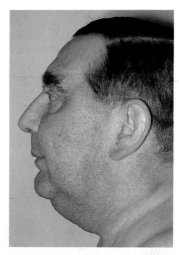

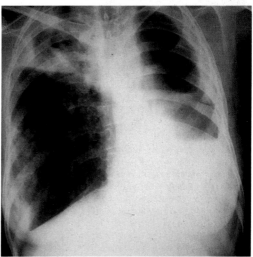

13 This 50-year-old woman with diabetes mellitus presented with a cough, night sweats and weight loss. She was found to have a low-grade fever and the chest X-ray illustrated. What is the likely diagnosis and what abnormalities are shown?

14

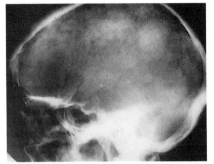

14 The X-ray shows diffuse mottling of the skull. Which of the following is likely to be the cause: multiple myeloma, secondary carcinoma, hyperparathyroidism, Paget's disease?

15

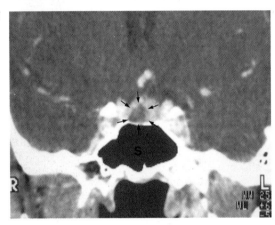

15 (a) This cranial CT scan after contrast was taken from a 30-year-old woman with a two-year history of secondary amenorrhoea and galactorrhoea. What does the scan show?

(b) Which of the following statements about a prolactinoma are correct?

(i) Prolactinomas are usually hypodense on CT scan after contrast.

(ii) Prolactinomas often arise as a result of prior oral contraceptive therapy.

(iii) Microprolactinomas are more common than macroprolactinomas.

(iv) A prolactin level of 1000 mU/l (normal level is < 340 mU/l) in the presence of a large tumour extending beyond the fossa suggests the presence of a 'pseudo-prolactinoma'.

(v) Prolactinomas are usually not radiosensitive.

16 (a) What condition is illustrated in this picture showing a 17-year-old girl who complained of swelling in the neck and of acne?

(b) Which of the following statements about this condition are true?

(i) Hyperplasia or neoplasia of the C-cells of the thyroid is involved.

(ii) Mucosal neuromas are seen in the eyelids, lips and tongue.

(iii) Peripheral neuropathy is common.

(iv) Phaeochromocytomas and parathyroid adenomas are seen.

(v) Ganglioneuromas of the bowel are associated.

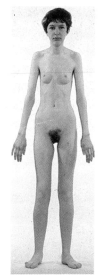

17 (a) This elderly woman is a diabetic. What pancreatic cause can you deduce for her diabetes?

(b) Which of the following pancreatic conditions may lead to diabetes:

(i) chronic pancreatitis,

(ii) haemochromatosis,

(iii) removal of an islet-cell tumour,

(iv) cystic fibrosis,

(v) mumps pancreatitis?

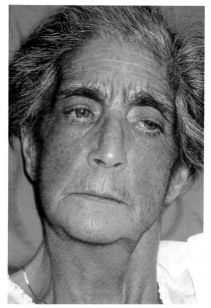

18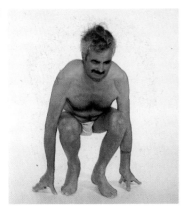

19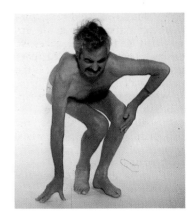

20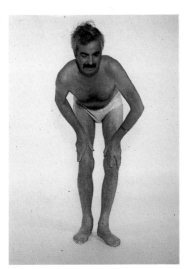

18–20 (a) What is wrong with this man?
(b) Which of the following endocrine conditions may be responsible: acromegaly, Cushing's syndrome, hypothyroidism, diabetes mellitus, Conn's syndrome?

21 (a) This 20-year-old man complained of difficulty in going upstairs and had noticed excessive bruising of his arms and legs over the previous 6 months. What is the most likely diagnosis?

(b) Which of the following investigations would be appropriate:

(i) 24-hour urinary free cortisol,
(ii) plasma ACTH at 0900 hours,
(iii) chest X-ray,
(iv) plasma thyroxine concentration,
(v) plasma electrolytes?

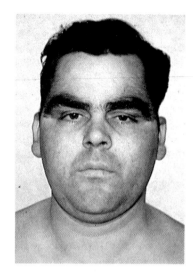

22 This 11-year-old child was 120 cm tall. On investigation, she was found to have the following abnormalities—a raised blood urea and creatinine, a low serum calcium and a raised phosphate level. Which of the following diagnoses fit the clinical picture: chronic renal failure, hypoparathyroidism, rickets, vitamin D intoxication?

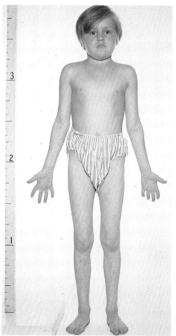

23

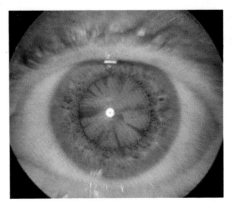

23 (a) What chronic complication of diabetes mellitus is illustrated here?
(b) Which of the following statements about this condition are correct?
  (i) They can occur in young patients.
  (ii) They are not usually bilateral.
  (iii) Poor metabolic control is associated.
  (iv) It does not occur in diabetes in old age.
  (v) The snowflake appearance is typical of diabetes.

24

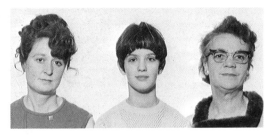

24 (a) This family group consists of a 35-year-old woman with Graves' disease, her 14-year-old daughter with lymphocytic thyroiditis, and her 70-year-old mother with myxoedema. What is the underlying type of disease in this family and what serological abnormality are they all likely to exhibit?
(b) Which of the following conditions are recognised associations of this variety of thyroid disease:
  (i) vitiligo,
  (ii) allergic alveolitis,
  (iii) pernicious anaemia,
  (iv) primary biliary cirrhosis,
  (v) bronchogenic carcinoma?

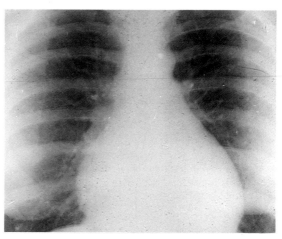

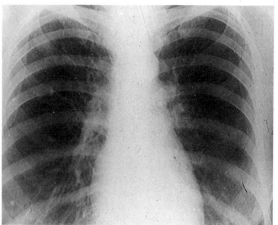

25, 26 (a) The chest X-ray in **25** was obtained from a 60-year-old woman who complained of lack of energy and shortness of breath. She was found to be clinically hypothyroid and responded to treatment with thyroxine 0.1 mg daily. Her chest X-ray 3 months later is shown in **26**. What condition do the X-rays illustrate?

(b) Which of the following complications are recognised associations of hypothyroidism:
    (i) ascites,
    (ii) uveal effusions,
    (iii) hydroceles,
    (iv) sinusitis,
    (v) inner ear effusions?

27

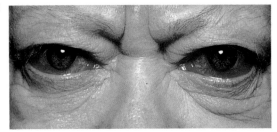

27 Which of the following eye signs of Graves' disease does this patient exhibit:
(i) lid retraction,
(ii) exophthalmos,
(iii) periorbital swelling,
(iv) ophthalmoplegia,
(v) conjunctival injection?

28

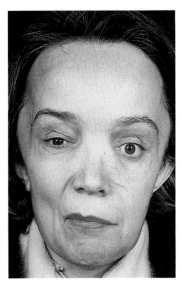

28 (a) This patient presented with left-sided facial weakness. What is the probable cause?
(b) Which of the following may also complicate the underlying disease:
(i) deafness
(ii) anosmia
(iii) Erb's paralysis
(iv) sciatica?

29, 30 (a) This 19-year-old boy presented with gross obesity and was mentally retarded. What is the likely diagnosis?

(b) Which of the following features are seen in this syndrome:

  (i) hyperphagia,
  (ii) retinitis pigmentosa,
  (iii) polydactyly,
  (iv) diabetes insipidus,
  (v) hypogonadism,
  (vi) short fourth metacarpals?

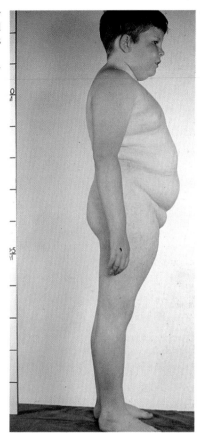

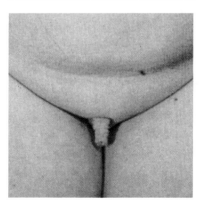

31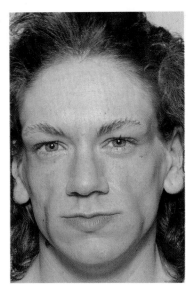

3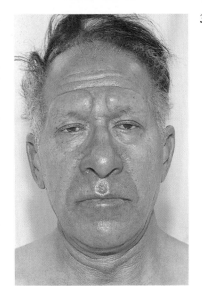

33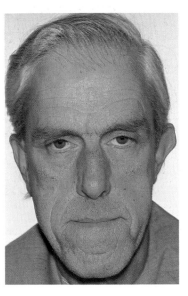

3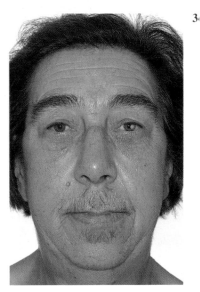

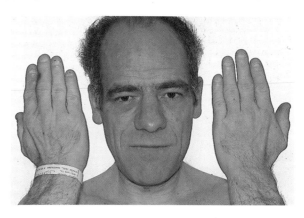

31–35 Match the pictures with these diagnoses: acromegaly, lipoatrophy, acromegaly, Hashimoto's disease, and hypothyroidism, normal variant.

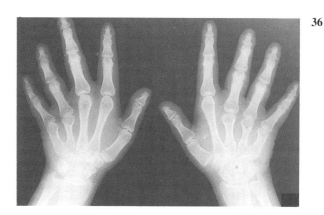

36 (a) What radiological abnormality is shown?
(b) Which of the following clinical features may be associated with this abnormality: webbing of the neck, tetany, exostoses, pathological fractures?

37

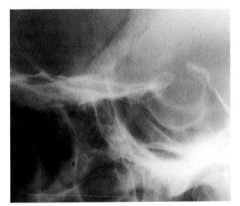

37 (a) This lateral skull X-ray is of a 24-year-old woman whose only complaint was of 4 years' valid infertility. She had a normal menstrual cycle. No abnormalities could be detected on examination. What does the skull X-ray show?

(b) Which of the following investigations would be relevant to this patient:
   (i) serum prolactin,
   (ii) measurement of the visual fields,
   (iii) ultrasound examination of the ovaries,
   (iv) chest X-ray,
   (v) karyotype examination of the patient's blood?

38

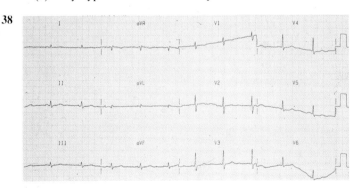

38 (a) What is the major abnormality shown on this electrocardiogram?
(b) Which of the following conditions may be associated with this abnormality:
   (i) Conn's syndrome,
   (ii) hypothyroidism,
   (iii) Addison's disease,
   (iv) hypoparathyroidism?

39 (a) What radiological abnormality is shown on the X-ray?
(b) Which of the following conditions may be associated with this finding: rickets, achondroplasia, Turner's syndrome, Klinefelter's syndrome?

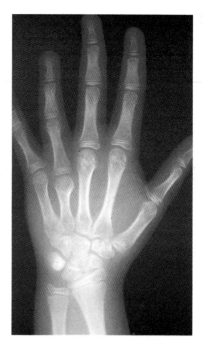

40 (a) Why was this 30-year-old woman's diabetes mellitus difficult to control?
(b) Which of the following statements about the patient's underlying condition are correct?

    (i) Weight gain excludes the diagnosis.

    (ii) Thirst is a not uncommon complaint.

    (iii) Increased appetite associated with loss of weight only occurs in this condition.

    (iv) Increased absorption of glucose is a feature.

    (v) Correction of the metabolic abnormality is followed by improved control of the associated diabetes.

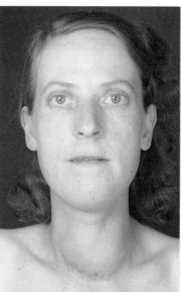

41

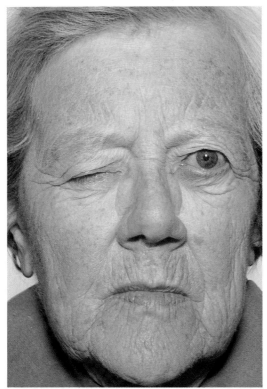

42

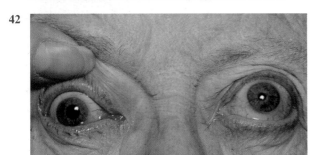

41, 42 What clinical features does this patient exhibit, and in a patient with known pituitary disease what do they imply?

43 This 12-year-old child presented with shortness of stature and was also noted to have thin skin, alopecia and severe arthritis. Which of the following diagnoses fit the clinical picture: pituitary dwarfism, hypothyroidism, progeria, polyostotic fibrous dysplasia?

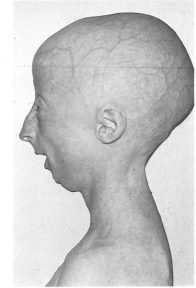

44 (a) This 15-year-old girl had been deaf since birth. She complained of increasing swelling in her neck and was found to have a moderate, soft, non-vascular goitre. She was clinically euthyroid. A brother was also deaf and had had a partial thyroidectomy for a non-toxic goitre. What is the likely diagnosis?

(b) Which of the following are recognised features of this condition:

   (i) autosomal recessive inheritance,

   (ii) a positive perchlorate discharge test indicating a thyroid organification defect,

   (iii) a tendency for the goitre to recur after partial thyroidectomy,

   (iv) an increased circulating level of monoiodotyrosine (MIT),

   (v) the combination of a raised serum thyroid-stimulating hormone (TSH), a low fT4 and a normal or raised fT3 level?

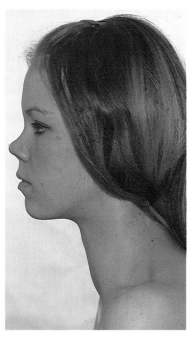

45

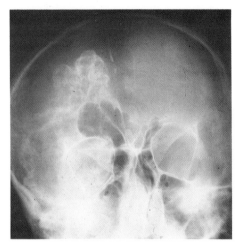

45 (a) What radiological abnormality is shown?
(b) Which of the following benign tumours may be associated with this lesion: meningioma, carcinoid syndrome, phaeochromocytoma, capillary haemangioma, fibrolipoma?

46

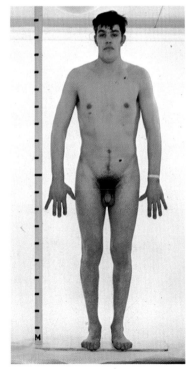

46 This man of 1.97 m height was referred with possible acromegaly and gigantism. Which of the following conditions fit the clinical picture:
(i) acromegaly and gigantism,
(ii) familial tall stature,
(iii) Klinefelter's syndrome,
(iv) congenital adrenal hyperplasia,
(v) XYY syndrome?

47 (a) This is the axilla of a 20-year-old, grossly obese girl who presented with diabetes mellitus. What is the lesion?

(b) Which of the following statements about this skin condition are true?

    (i) It is asymptomatic.

    (ii) It progresses to malignant melanoma.

    (iii) It tends to be associated with malignancy.

    (iv) It has a tendency to resolve spontaneously.

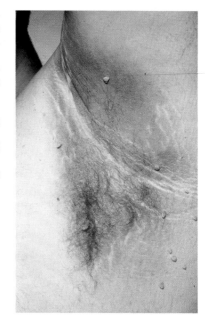

48 The child on the left, with growth retardation and normal skeletal proportions, is standing next to an age- and sex-matched control. Which of the following endocrine conditions may be responsible: hypothyroidism, hyperthyroidism, hypoadrenalism, Cushing's syndrome?

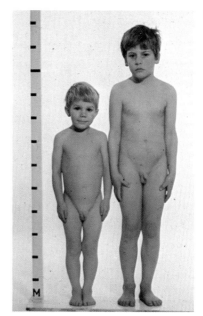

49

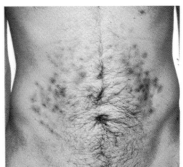

50

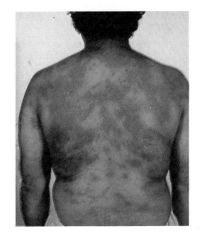

51

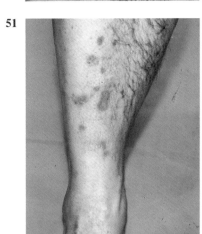

52

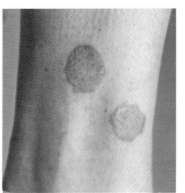

53

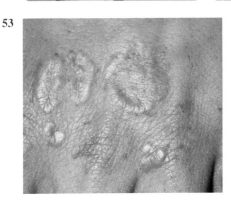

49–53 Match these clinical pictures of dermatological disease in diabetes with the following diagnoses: granuloma annulare, necrobiosis lipoidica, acanthosis nigricans, diabetic dermopathy, furunculosis.

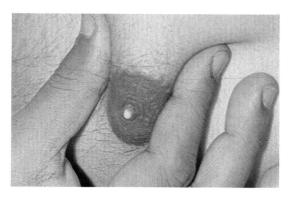

54 (a) This 25-year-old man complained of milky secretion from the breasts of one year's duration. There was no gynaecomastia and no other abnormalities could be detected on clinical examination. What condition is illustrated here and would you expect the prolactin (PRL) level to be elevated?

(b) Which of the following statements about this condition are true?

(i) It is not usually associated with gynaecomastia.

(ii) Gynaecomastia is best detected by picking up the breast tissue between the finger and thumb.

(iii) Gynaecomastia generally results from oestrogen/androgen imbalance.

(iv) Increased oestrogen ingestion may enhance PRL secretion.

(v) It often does not accompany a raised PRL.

55

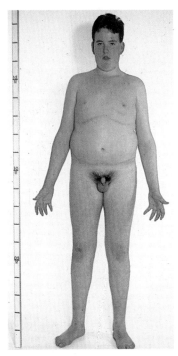

55 (a) This 18-year-old male presented with sexual immaturity. He was found to have very small testes and to have an XXY chromosome constitution. What is the diagnosis?

(b) Which of the following statements are true of this condition?

(i) Plasma testosterone levels are reduced.

(ii) Plasma gonadotrophin levels are raised.

(iii) Plasma cortisol levels are reduced.

(iv) Plasma growth hormone level is raised.

56

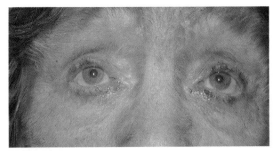

56 (a) What physical sign is illustrated?

(b) Which of the following conditions may be responsible: acromegaly, anorexia nervosa, carcinoma of the bronchus, Cushing's syndrome?

57 This 21-year-old woman presented with primary amenorrhoea and it was noted on physical examination that she was anosmic. Which of the following diagnoses fit the clinical picture: Turner's syndrome, prolactinoma, Kallmann's syndrome, congenital adrenal hyperplasia?

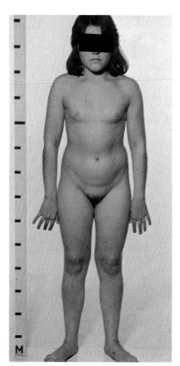

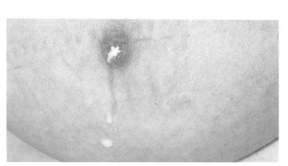

58 (a) What condition is illustrated here?

(b) Which of the following investigations might be helpful in identifying the cause:

    (i) serum calcium,   (iv) lateral skull X-ray,

    (ii) serum thyroxine,   (v) plasma cortisol?

    (iii) blood glucose,

59

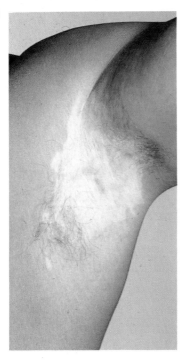

59 (a) This 30-year-old man complained of loss of pigmentation in the left axilla. What condition is illustrated here?

(b) Which of the following statements about this condition are likely to be correct?

(i) The condition could have been present from birth.

(ii) There is likely to be some depigmentation in the other axilla.

(iii) It is associated with other organ-specific autoimmune diseases which should be sought.

(iv) There may also be increased pigmentation of the hair.

(v) The depigmentation tends to be surrounded by an area of increased pigmentation.

60

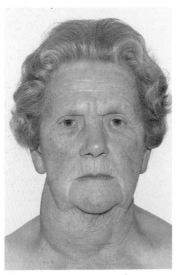

60 (a) This 70-year-old woman attended clinic complaining of a swelling in the neck. This had first developed 3 months earlier and had rapidly increased in size. On examination she had a large, hard mass in the right side of the neck without lymphadenopathy, which was displacing the trachea to the left and which moved on swallowing. What is the likely diagnosis?

(b) Which of the following features would make you strongly suspect malignancy in this condition:

(i) asymmetry,

(ii) lymphadenopathy,

(iii) rapid, painful increase in size,

(iv) hoarseness,

(v) fixation of the mass to skin and deep tissue?

61 (a) What condition is illustrated in this 50-year-old diabetic woman?
(b) Which of the following may be associated with this condition: hyperlipidaemia, subcutaneous xanthomas, hepatomegaly, splenomegaly, acanthosis nigricans?

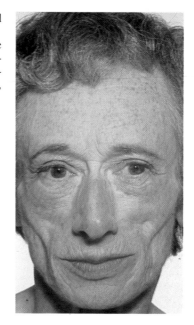

62 (a) What procedure is being carried out in this illustration?
(b) Which of the following statements about this procedure are correct?

(i) It is a very useful diagnostic test.

(ii) It is not possible to separate follicular adenomas from follicular carcinomas by this technique.

(iii) It is useful to confirm the presence of a thyroid cyst.

(iv) It clearly separates all malignant from benign lesions.

(v) It is painful to the patient who is best premedicated with intravenous diazepam.

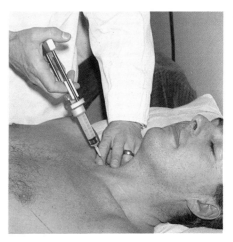

63

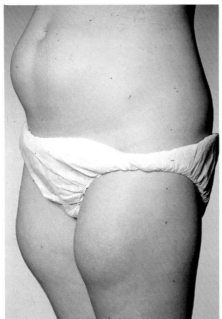

64

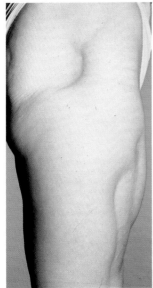

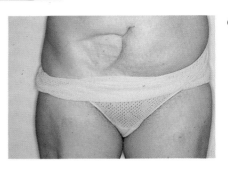

65

63–65 (a) What complications of insulin therapy are shown?
(b) How may these be prevented?

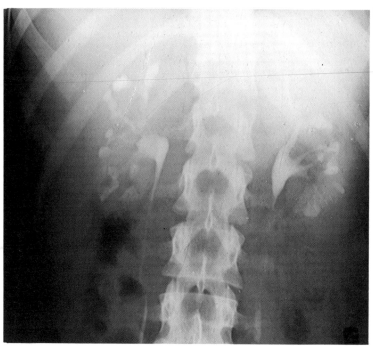

66 (a) This intravenous pyelogram was obtained from a 50-year-old, insulin-dependent diabetic with pyelonephritis. What abnormalities does it show?

(b) Which of the following complications may be seen in a diabetic with secondary renal disease:
  (i) hypertension,
  (ii) necrotising papillitis,
  (iii) diabetic glomerulonephritis,
  (iv) a nephrotic syndrome,
  (v) IgA nephropathy?

67

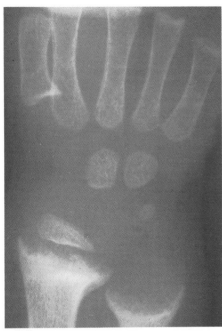

67 (a) What abnormality is demonstrated and what is the cause?

(b) Which of the following biochemical abnormalities are likely to be present: low serum calcium, low serum phosphate, low urinary hydroxyproline, low serum alkaline phosphatase?

68

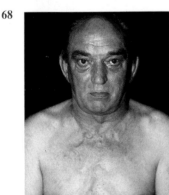
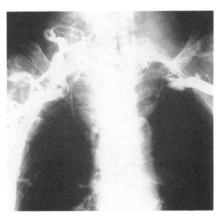

68, 69 (a) This 50-year-old man complained of headaches and swelling of the face along with difficulty in swallowing. He had an audible stridor. What is the likely diagnosis?

(b) Which of the following causes should be regarded as likely to be responsible for this condition: retrosternal goitre, bronchogenic carcinoma, lymphoma, leukaemia, hypernephroma?

70 (a) This patient complained of polyuria and weight loss, and had a fasting blood glucose of 12 mmol/l. What is the likely diagnosis?

(b) Which of the following statements about this condition are correct?

(i) Polyuria and nocturia may occur in the absence of hyperglycaemia.

(ii) Cortisol enhances gluconeogenesis.

(iii) Cortisol enhances peripheral glucose utilisation.

(iv) Carbohydrate intolerance is found in about 90% with this syndrome.

(v) The hyperglycaemia is easily controlled by oral hypoglycaemic drugs.

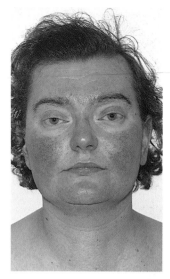

71 This 17-year-old boy complained of swelling of the breasts. He was tall, of eunuchoid proportions, had bilateral gynaecomastia and small, firm pea-sized testes, of 0.5 ml volume. Which of the following statements about this condition are true?

(i) It is normally associated with a 47XXY karyotype.

(ii) The Leydig cells in the testes may appear histologically normal or hyperplastic.

(iii) The plasma testosterone level may be normal.

(iv) The serum luteinizing hormone (LH) level is invariably raised but the follicle-stimulating hormone (FSH) level is normal.

(v) Caution must be exercised when contemplating androgen medication in such patients.

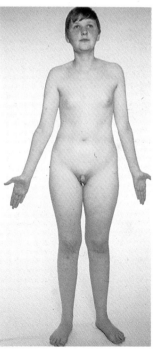

72

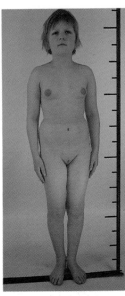

72 This 16-year-old girl presented with short stature, primary amenorrhoea, immature genitalia and pigmented nipples, and hypopituitarism.
(a) What clinical conditions should be suspected in this girl?
(b) What clinical features does she exhibit? List the relevant tests.

73

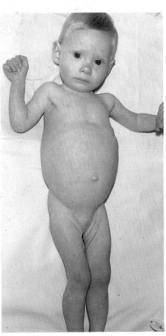

73 This child, with failure to thrive, had linear height below the third percentile for age. What clinical features are shown and what is the probable diagnosis?

74 This radiograph shows a translucent area in the upper tibia of an 18-year-old female with irregular pigmentation and a history of precocious puberty. Which of the following diagnoses is the most probable: congenital adrenal hyperplasia, neurofibromatosis, polyostotic fibrous dysplasia, hyperparathyroidism?

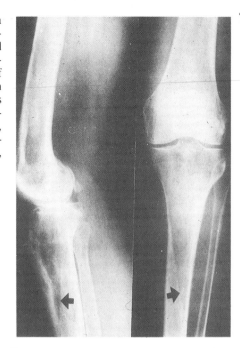

75 (a) What diabetic complication is illustrated here?
(b) Which of the following statements about this condition are true?

   (i) Affected patients often complain of intermittent claudication.
   (ii) Adjacent infection is rarely a problem.
   (iii) X-rays rarely reveal an underlying osteitis.
   (iv) Local amputation can yield good results.
   (v) There is no value in advising such patients to give up smoking.

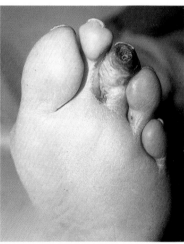

76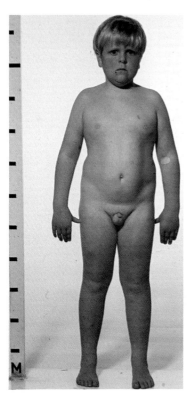

76 (a) This 10-year-old boy has a height of 1.15 m (below the third percentile) and was brought to his general practitioner because of shortness of stature. Does this condition warrant further investigation, and what diagnosis is it important to exclude or confirm?
(b) What clinical features does this boy exhibit which might help to point to a clinical diagnosis?

77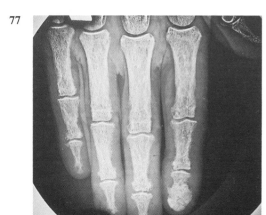

77 (a) What lesions are shown in the X-ray?
(b) Which of the following investigations might be helpful in identifying the cause:
  (i) serum calcium,
  (ii) serum thyroxine,
  (iii) chest X-ray,
  (iv) blood glucose?

78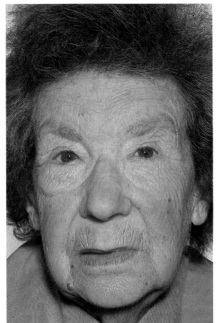

79

80

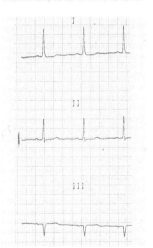

78–80 (a) What condition is illustrated in this 80-year-old woman (**78**) who complained of loss of energy, tingling of the fingers, and feeling the cold?

(b) These electrocardiograms were obtained before (**79**) and after (**80**) appropriate medication for her condition. Which of the following are recognised electrocardiographic features of this condition:
  (i) bradycardia,
  (ii) low voltage P waves,
  (iii) sinus arrhythmia,
  (iv) inverted T waves,
  (v) increased voltage R waves?

81

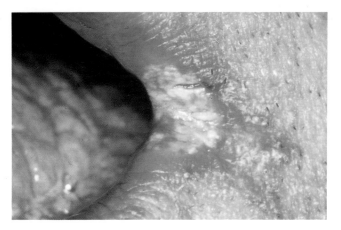

81 (a) What condition is illustrated in this diabetic patient?
(b) Which of the following disorders are known to be complicated by this condition:
  (i) AIDS (HIV infection),
  (ii) anticoagulant therapy with warfarin,
  (iii) oral contraceptive medication,
  (iv) corticosteroid therapy,
  (v) broad-spectrum antibiotic therapy?

82

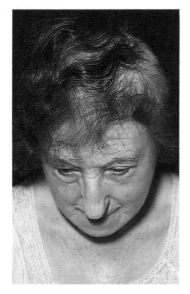

82 (a) This woman complained of scalp hair loss, but was otherwise well. What is the likely diagnosis?
(b) Which of the following statements about this disorder are correct?

  (i) It is commonly precipitated by emotional upset.

  (ii) Spontaneous resolution is common.

  (iii) It is associated with psoriasis.

  (iv) It is associated with clinical and/or serological evidence of thyroid autoimmunity.

  (v) It responds readily to therapy.

83 (a) The illustration shows a 12-year-old girl. Median height for this age is 1.47 m. What two physical signs are shown in the photograph in addition to the shortness of stature?
(b) What is the probable diagnosis?
(c) What is the mode of inheritance?

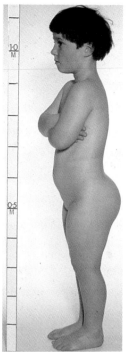

84 (a) This 15-year-old boy presented with swelling of the breasts. He was noted to be grossly obese and mentally retarded. What diagnosis should be considered?
(b) Which of the following statements about this condition are true?
(i) The apparent gynaecomastia is largely due to fat deposition.
(ii) The obesity is due to hyperphagia of hypothalamic origin.
(iii) Mental retardation is a feature of the syndrome.
(iv) Diabetes insipidus is a common complication.
(v) The patients have rather large hands and feet.

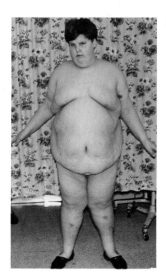

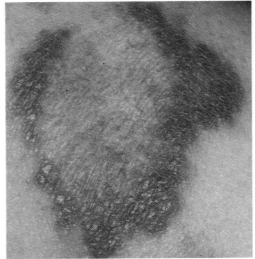

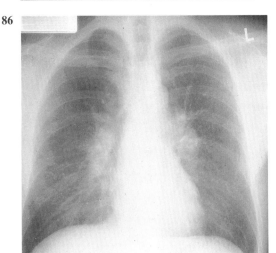

85, 86 (a) This skin lesion and the chest X-ray are from the same patient. What is the diagnosis? (b) Which of the following abnormalities may be associated with this condition: hyperuricaemia, hyperglycaemia, hypercholesterolaemia, hypercalcaemia?

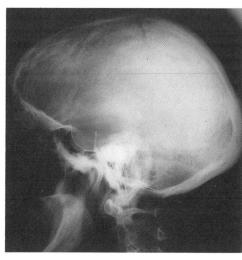

87 (a) This skull X-ray was taken from a woman who had been previously diagnosed as having the Zollinger–Ellison syndrome and who had been cured by removal of a gastrin-secreting adenoma from her duodenum. What abnormality is shown on the X-ray and what familial condition should be considered?

(b) Which of the following statements about this condition are correct?

(i) It is recessively inherited.

(ii) Phaeochromocytomas are an important part of the syndrome.

(iii) It should be considered in all patients with pituitary, parathyroid, or pancreatic islet-cell tumours.

(iv) If a lesion is found in more than one organ, all first-degree relatives should be screened with skull X-ray, fasting blood sugar and serum calcium estimations.

(v) The tumours responsible are invariably benign.

88

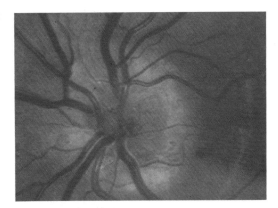

89

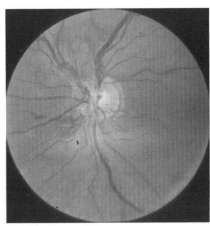

88, 89 What features of diabetic retinopathy are featured in these retinal photographs?

90

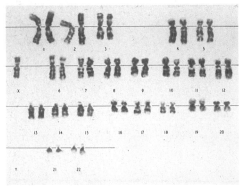

90 (a) What chromosomal abnormality is shown? (b) Which of the following statements are likely to be true in a patient with this chromosomal constitution?

(i) The patient will be phenotypically female.

(ii) Clitoral hypertrophy will develop at puberty.

(iii) Breast development is poor.

(iv) Facial hirsutism is common.

91 (a) What condition is this patient likely to be suffering from?
(b) Which of the following eye signs does she exhibit:
- (i) lid retraction,
- (ii) exophthalmos,
- (iii) periorbital swelling,
- (iv) congestive ophthalmopathy,
- (v) ophthalmoplegia?

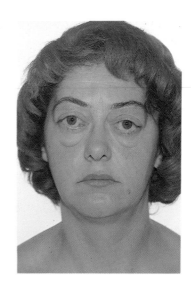

92 The X-ray shows radio-opaque renal calculi. Which of the following endocrine/metabolic conditions may be responsible: renal hypercalciuria, primary hyperparathyroidism, renal tubular acidosis, cystinuria?

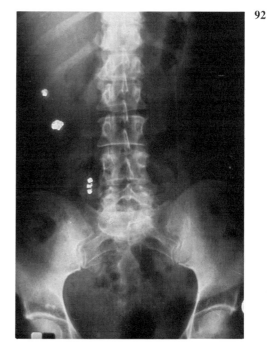

93 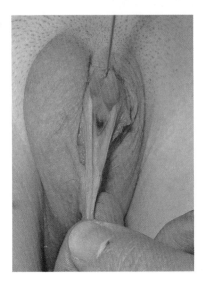 (a) What abnormalities are shown in the photograph?
(b) Which of the following syndromes may be associated with these abnormalities: Ullrich–Turner syndrome, congenital adrenal hyperplasia, Klinefelter's syndrome, Reifenstein's syndrome?

94 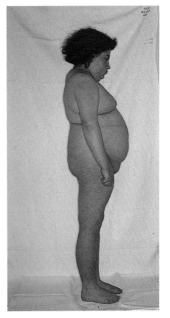 This 12-year-old child has been referred for investigation of shortness of stature. Which of the following endocrine conditions should be considered in the differential diagnosis: Cushing's syndrome, Conn's syndrome, congenital adrenal hyperplasia, phaeochromocytoma?

95 (a) What physical sign is seen in this middle-aged male?

(b) Which of the following endocrine abnormalities may be associated with this sign:

    (i) acromegaly,

    (ii) Cushing's syndrome,

    (iii) hypopituitarism,

    (iv) Addison's disease,

    (v) Klinefelter's syndrome?

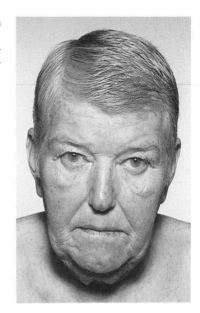

96 (a) This 50-year-old woman complained of increased sweating, and swelling in her neck. What is the likely diagnosis?

(b) Which of the following statements about thyroid disease in this condition are true?

    (i) Goitre occurs in about 20% of patients.

    (ii) Most patients are euthyroid.

    (iii) The most common cause of thyroid enlargement is a nodular goitre.

    (iv) The goitre may well be due to increased circulating levels of somatomedin-C.

    (v) Thyroid hormone binding protein abnormalities are common.

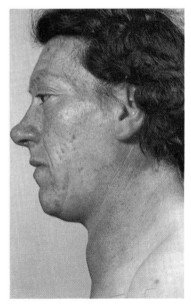

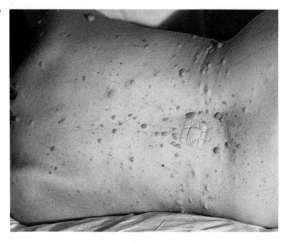

97 (a) What condition is shown?
(b) Which of the following disorders may be associated with this condition: phaeochromocytoma, Cushing's syndrome, medullary carcinoma of the thyroid, bronchial carcinoma, carcinoid syndrome, hypernephroma?

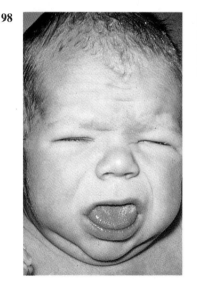

98 This 2-week-old child was diagnosed as having neonatal hypothyroidism as a result of a Guthrie screening test at 8 days. Which of the following statements is likely to be correct?

(i) The best screening test is measurement of free thyroxine.

(ii) The prevalence in western countries is of the order of 1 in 3500 live births.

(iii) Neonatal hypothyroidism due to pituitary TSH deficiency is as common as that due to primary thyroid disease.

(iv) It can rarely result from transplacental passage of TSH-receptor blocking antibodies.

(v) It presents with clear physical signs which can be used as the basis of diagnosis.

99 (a) This 60-year-old woman has a long-standing swelling in the neck which has increased in size recently. What condition is she likely to exhibit?

(b) Which of the following statements are likely to be correct?

(i) She shows eye signs of Graves' disease.

(ii) Malignancy is a likely explanation.

(iii) Iodine deficiency could have contributed to the development of the goitre.

(iv) Administration of iodine would help in the resolution of her goitre.

(v) She is likely to have circulating thyrotrophin-receptor antibodies.

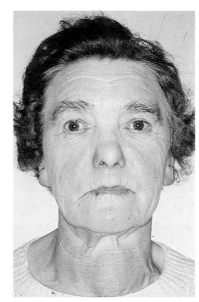

100 (a) What is the probable diagnosis in this patient?

(b) Which of the following symptoms are likely to be present: obesity, cold intolerance, oedema, back pain?

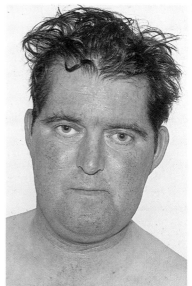

101

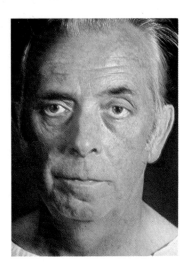

101 (a) This middle-aged man complained of attacks of flushing and chronic, profuse, watery diarrhoea. What condition may he be suffering from?

(b) Which of the following abnormalities accompany this condition:

(i) dehydration,

(ii) hypoglycaemia,

(iii) hyperchlorhydria,

(iv) elevated levels of vasoactive intestinal peptide (VIP),

(v) elevated levels of pancreatic polypeptide (PP)?

102

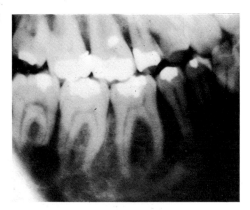

102 This X-ray was reported as showing absence of the lamina dura. Which of the following abnormalities are likely to be associated with this finding: raised serum calcium, lowered serum calcium, raised plasma cortisol, raised blood glucose?

103 (a) This child was brought to the clinic on account of shortness of stature, increased bowing of the legs, and thickening of the wrists and ankles. What is the probable diagnosis? (b) Which of the following disorders may be responsible:
  (i) gluten-sensitive enteropathy,
  (ii) renal tubular acidosis,
  (iii) hypoparathyroidism,
  (iv) pituitary failure,
  (v) epilepsy?

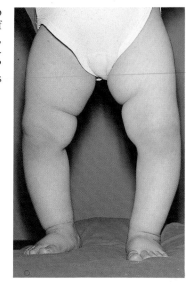

103

104 (a) This 45-year-old woman was found to have glycosuria on routine testing of the urine and a fasting blood glucose level of 10 mmol/l. What is the likely diagnosis?
(b) Which of the following statements about her condition are true?
  (i) It is characterised by marked insulin insensitivity.
  (ii) Post-mortem studies have shown a 20–30% decrease in B-cell mass.
  (iii) Genetic factors play a significant part in its development.
  (iv) Islet-cell antibodies are usually present.
  (v) It generally presents over the age of 40.

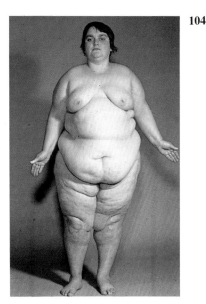

104

105

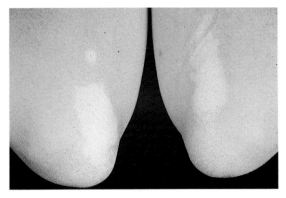

105 (a) What skin condition is illustrated?
(b) Which of the following conditions may be associated with this disorder: Addison's disease, congenital adrenal hyperplasia, phaeochromocytoma, Conn's syndrome, carcinoid syndrome?

106

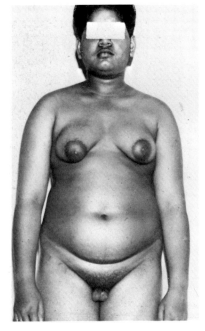

106 This patient was considered phenotypically male until the age of puberty when breast development occurred. He was found to have hypospadias and a 46XX/XY mosaic on karyotyping. Which of the following diagnoses fits the clinical picture: congenital adrenal hyperplasia, Reifenstein's syndrome, true hermaphroditism, Ullrich–Turner syndrome?

107 (a) What physical sign is illustrated?

(b) Which of the following conditions may be responsible:
  (i) polycystic ovary syndrome,
  (ii) Cushing's syndrome,
  (iii) congenital adrenal hyperplasia,
  (iv) anorexia nervosa?

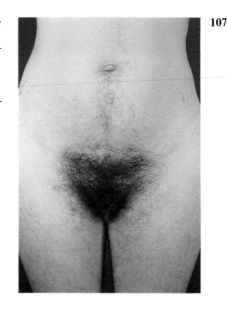

108 (a) What lesion is shown in the X-ray?

(b) With which metabolic disorders of bone may this lesion be associated: Paget's disease of bone, hyperparathyroidism, osteomalacia, osteogenesis imperfecta, polyostotic fibrous dysplasia?

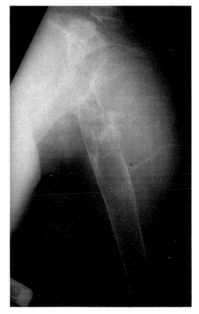

109

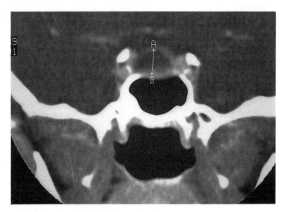

110

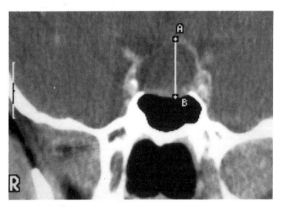

109, 110 (a) These CT scans were taken after contrast before pregnancy and in the third trimester in a 25-year-old woman who initially presented with amenorrhoea and galactorrhoea and a prolactin level of 1500 mU/l. What do the scans show?

(b) Which of the following statements about this condition in pregnancy are correct?

(i) The lesion may expand during pregnancy.

(ii) Expansion usually presents with increasing headache, nausea, vomiting and a visual field defect.

(iii) The field defect is characteristically a homonymous hemianopia.

(iv) Patients who become pregnant should have monthly visual field checks.

(v) Expansion during pregnancy should on no account be treated with bromocriptine because of the drug's teratogenic effects.

111 This normotensive 10-year-old post-pubertal boy was found to have raised plasma ACTH and raised 17-α-OH progesterone. Which of the following diagnoses fit the clinical picture:

(i) Cushing's syndrome,
(ii) Leydig cell tumour of the testes,
(iii) congenital adrenal hyperplasia —21-hydroxylase defect,
(iv) congenital adrenal hyperplasia —11-hydroxylase defect?

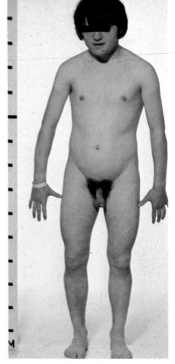

112 (a) This 25-year-old man complained of swelling of the neck of 6 months' duration. A known asthmatic, he required systemic steroid medication. He was clinically euthyroid and had a large, soft, non-vascular goitre. What diagnosis should be strongly considered in his case?

(b) Which of the following statements about goitres in men are true?

(i) Goitres are as common in men as in women.
(ii) The cause of a goitre is usually apparent in a man.
(iii) Autoimmune thyroid disease should be considered if a goitre is firm and finely nodular.
(iv) Iodine deficiency goitres are common in men in the UK.
(v) Iodides are one of the most common goitrogens.

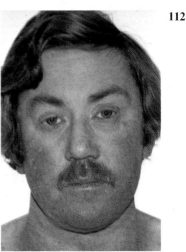

113

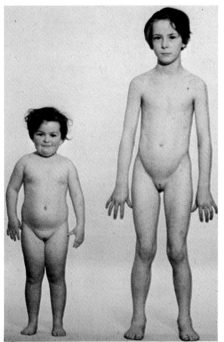

113 These children are both 9 years old. The child on the left is well below the third percentile for height for her age and was found to have retarded bone age. Which of the following investigations may be helpful in determining the cause for the growth retardation:

(i) glucose tolerance test,
(ii) arginine test,
(iii) serum thyrotrophin,
(iv) serum thyroxine,
(v) skull X-ray?

114

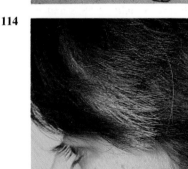

114 (a) What physical sign is shown in the illustration?

(b) Which of the following conditions may be associated with this sign:

(ii) diabetes mellitus,
(ii) Cushing's syndrome,
(iii) Addison's disease,
(iv) Turner's syndrome,
(v) polycystic ovary syndrome?

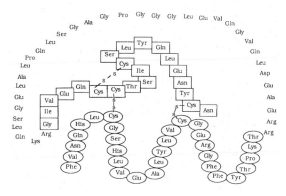

115 This figure shows the structure of human pro-insulin. Which of the following statements about insulin are correct?

(i) The insulin gene is located on the long arm of chromosome 11.

(ii) It consists of 135 base pairs, and is composed of 3 exons and 2 introns.

(iii) Proinsulin is produced from the mature mRNA and is transported to the Golgi apparatus where it is cleaved to insulin and C-peptide.

(iv) Insulin has a molecular weight of 5808 and it contains 51 amino acids.

(v) Glucose is the major stimulus for insulin release from its storage granules.

116 This patient presented with gynae-comastia and small testes and a diagnosis of Klinefelter's syndrome was made. Which of the following statements are true of this condition?

(i) Only males are affected.

(ii) All patients are sterile.

(iii) The chromosome constitution is XYY.

(iv) There is an increased risk of carcinoma of the breast.

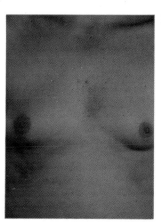

116

117

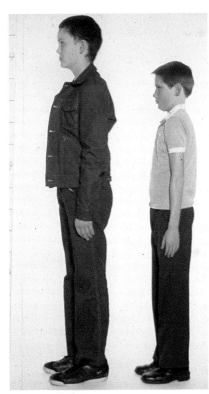

117 The 11-year-old boy on the left is shown with an age-matched control. Which of the following investigations are required to confirm or refute a diagnosis of gigantism:

(i) measurement of growth hormone (GH) levels during a glucose tolerance test,

(ii) measurement of GH levels during hypoglycaemia,

(iii) measurement of GH levels after arginine administration,

(iv) skull X-ray?

118

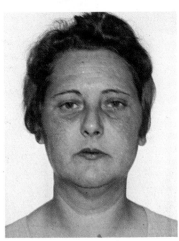

118 This caucasian patient had had a bilateral total adrenalectomy for Cushing's disease five years previously and had noted increased pigmentation of the skin over the previous year, associated with increasingly severe temporal headaches. What is the likely diagnosis? (b) Which of the following are regular features of this condition:

(i) a high plasma ACTH level,

(ii) high plasma cortisol levels,

(iii) marked deposition of melanin in the skin,

(iv) an enlarged pituitary fossa,

(v) diabetes insipidus?

119 This 50-year-old man had been referred with a possible diagnosis of Cushing's syndrome. In which of the following conditions may this appearance also be seen: hypothyroidism, depression, simple obesity, chronic alcoholism, essential hypertension?

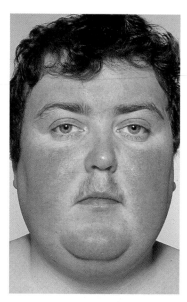

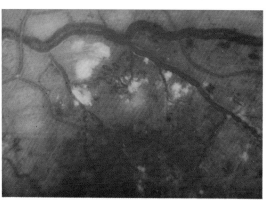

120 (a) What clinical disorder is likely to underlie this retinal photograph?
(b) Which of the following abnormalities are illustrated here:
  (i) microaneurysms,
  (ii) choroidoretinitis,
  (iii) hard exudates,
  (iv) venous dilatation,
  (v) pre-retinal haemorrhages?

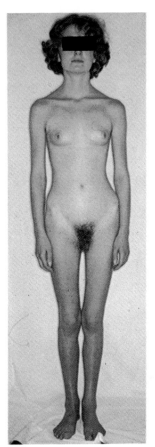

121 This patient was referred on account of secondary amenorrhoea and weight loss. Investigation revealed low circulating gonadotrophin levels, plasma growth hormone was high (but showed suppression during a glucose tolerance test) and plasma cortisol levels were high. All other endocrine function tests were normal. Which of the following diagnoses fit the clinical picture: acromegaly, Cushing's syndrome, premature ovarian failure, anorexia nervosa?

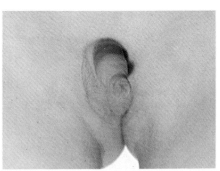

122 An empty scrotum in a 9-year-old boy is shown. Which of the following statements are likely to be true?

(i) Undescended testes will descend at puberty without treatment.

(ii) Undescended testes occur in approximately 1% of 9-year-old boys.

(iii) There is a greater risk of malignancy in undescended testes.

(iv) Orchidopexy should be carried out in children if the testes do not descend after treatment with human chorionic gonadotrophin (hCG).

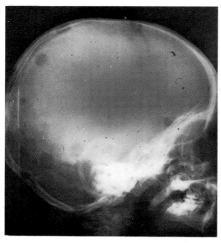

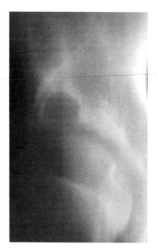

123, 124 (a) These X-rays are taken from a 10-year-old boy who developed polyuria and polydipsia and complained of headaches and shortness of stature. What is the likely diagnosis?
(b) Which of the following statements about this condition are true?
  (i) It affects adults as well as children.
  (ii) It is usually a relatively benign disease.
  (iii) Spontaneous pneumothorax may be a presenting sign of this condition.
  (iv) Lung infiltration is not uncommon.
  (v) Polyuria and polydipsia is a common presenting sign.

125 (a) What abnormality is seen in these external genitalia of an 18-year-old phenotypic female?
(b) Which of the following clinical features may be associated with this abnormality:
  (i) hirsutism,
  (ii) shortness of stature,
  (iii) hypertension,
  (iv) oedema?

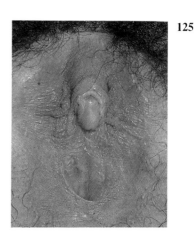

126

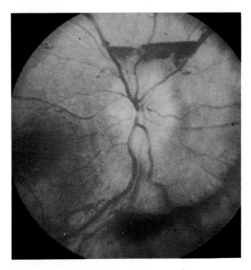

127

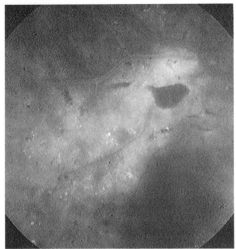

126, 127 (a) Name two conditions from which the haemorrhages in these retinal photographs could have resulted.
(b) Which of the following changes are shown:
    (i) subhyaloid haemorrhages,
    (ii) papilloedema,
    (iii) microaneurysms,
    (iv) hard exudates,
    (v) dilated veins?

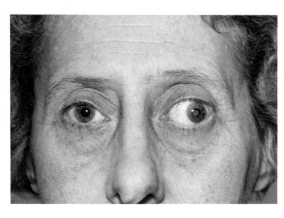

128 This 55-year-old woman was referred to an endocrinologist because her general practitioner had noticed that her left eye was unduly prominent during a routine check up. She had no complaints related to the eye and felt well. There were no other physical signs. Which of the following statements are true?

    (i) She has a lateral strabismus and therefore has a sixth nerve palsy.

    (ii) Her visual acuity in the left eye may well be diminished.

    (iii) She shows typical eye signs of Graves' disease.

    (iv) Examination of the left fundus could help to provide an explanation for her problem.

    (v) Appropriate treatment will resolve the prominence of the eye and improve her visual acuity.

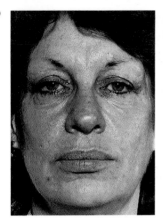 **129**

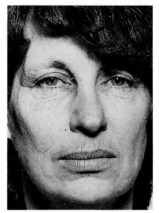 **130**

129, 130 (a) Provide two explanations for these illustrations.
(b) Which of the following criteria for a cure of acromegaly are true?
   (i) A marked reduction of the size of the hands and feet and reduction of soft-tissue swelling particularly of the face is evident.
   (ii) The growth hormone (GH) level should suppress to < 1.0 mU/l during a standard glucose tolerance test.
   (iii) There should be no GH response to thyrotrophin-releasing hormone (TRH).
   (iv) The GH level should rise in response to gonadotrophin-releasing hormone (GnRH).

131

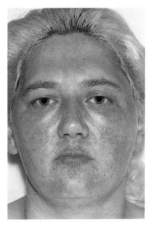

131 (a) This 50-year-old woman complained of frequent attacks of facial flushing and sweating each lasting for a few minutes. What is the likely diagnosis?
(b) Which of the following statements about this condition are true?
   (i) The flushes may commence before menstruation has ceased.
   (ii) The flushes nearly always cease in the first year after the menopause.
   (iii) They are usually associated with lowered circulating levels of 17 ß-oestradiol.
   (iv) The serum follicle-stimulating hormone (FSH) level remains normal.
   (v) They respond promptly to appropriate oestrogen medication.

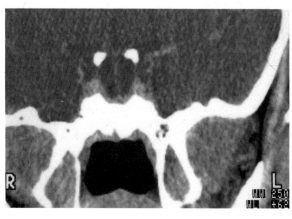

132

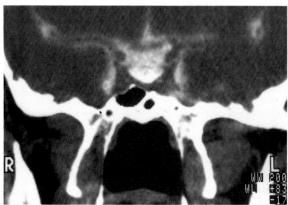

133

132, 133 (a) What do these CT scans show, and what condition do they illustrate?

(b) Which of the following statements about this condition are correct?

(i) The pituitary fossa is often enlarged on skull X-ray.

(ii) In most instances it does not result from a pituitary tumour.

(iii) The syndrome may be a late sequel of benign intracranial hypertension.

(iv) Pituitary hormone levels are usually normal in such patients.

(v) The most common cause is a congenital deficiency in the diaphragm sellae.

(vi) No treatment is required.

134

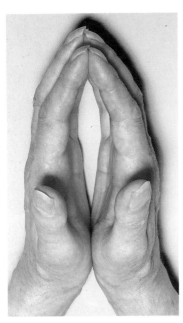

134 (a) These are the hands of a 40-year-old man with insulin-dependent diabetes. What is illustrated?

(b) Which of the following statements about this condition are true?

(i) It is more common in insulin-dependent diabetics.

(ii) It is often associated with a peripheral neuropathy.

(iii) It tends to occur in patients whose diabetes is poorly controlled.

(iv) It is not associated with Dupuytren's contracture.

(v) It is believed to result from abnormal glycosylation of collagen.

135

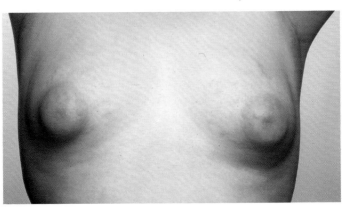

135 Breast development in an 8-year-old girl was associated with other pubertal changes. Which of the following conditions may lead to precocious puberty:

(i) Addison's disease,
(ii) hypothyroidism,
(iii) diabetes mellitus,

(iv) diabetes insipidus,
(v) germinoma of the pineal region?

136 (a) The enlarged lower leg of a 66-year-old man is shown. What is the probable diagnosis?

(b) Which of the following statements are true of this condition?

(i) The bone lesions only occur in the limb bones.

(ii) Men are more frequently affected than women.

(iii) The disorder is most frequent on the African continent.

(iv) Bone pain is characteristic of this disorder.

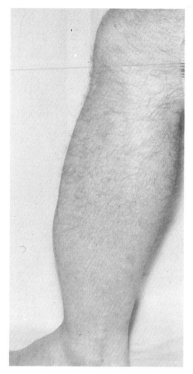

137 A dentist observed this abnormality in the buccal cavity and referred the patient to a physician.

(a) What possible diagnosis did the dentist consider?

(b) What are the key investigations to confirm or refute this diagnosis?

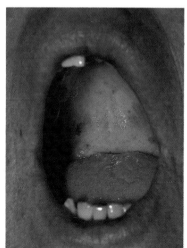

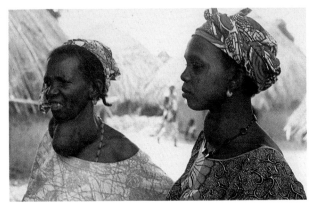

138 (a) These African women were noted to have swellings in their necks but had no complaints related to these. What is the likely diagnosis?

(b) Which of the following statements about this condition are correct?

(i) Iodine deficiency is the most likely cause.

(ii) Occasionally goitrogens may be involved.

(iii) Most adult patients are clinically euthyroid.

(iv) Endemic cretinism only occurs in areas of severe iodine deficiency.

(v) Intravenous iodine is the prophylaxis of choice.

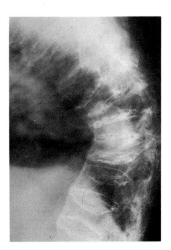

139 (a) Describe the radiological abnormalities shown.

(b) Which of the following disorders are likely to be associated with these abnormalities: hypothyroidism, premature ovarian failure, Cushing's syndrome, medullary carcinoma of the thyroid?

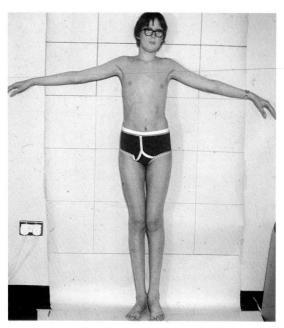

140 (a) This boy presented with tall stature and was found to have a finger tip to finger tip measurement 10 cm greater than his height. He was also noted to have abnormally long fingers and toes and a high arched palate. His growth hormone levels suppressed normally during a glucose tolerance test. What is the probable diagnosis?

(b) Which of the following somatic abnormalities may also be present:

    (i) coarctation of the aorta,
    (ii) aortic aneurysm,
    (iii) pectus excavatum,
    (iv) dislocation of the lens,
    (v) optic atrophy,
    (vi) deafness?

141

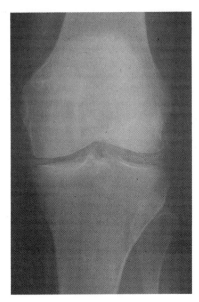

141 (a) This X-ray of the knee shows calcification of the menisci (chondrocalcinosis). What joint symptoms is this patient likely to experience?
(b) Which of the following metabolic disorders may be responsible:
    (i) hyperuricaemia,
    (ii) hyperparathyroidism,
    (iii) haemochromatosis,
    (iv) Wilson's disease?

142

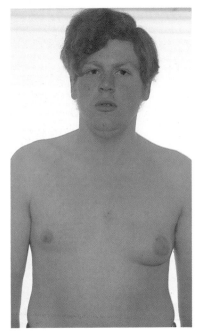

142 (a) This 16-year-old boy complained of bilateral tender swelling of the breasts of 6 months' duration. What is the likely diagnosis?
(b) Which of the following statements about this condition are true?
    (i) It is a common occurrence in normal boys.
    (ii) It is not usually tender.
    (iii) It usually remits spontaneously.
    (iv) It rarely causes any significant embarrassment.
    (v) If it persists surgical mastectomy may be indicated.

143 This man presented with increasing pigmentation following bilateral adrenalectomy for Cushing's disease (Nelson's syndrome). Which of the following statements are true of this condition: ACTH levels are raised, cortisol levels are raised, muscle weakness is common, skin fragility is increased?

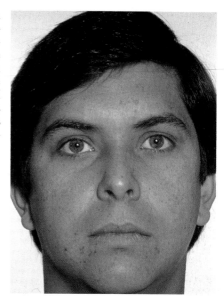

143

144 This 16-year-old boy presented with delayed puberty and shortness of stature. The penis, although small, was otherwise normal but the testes were impalpable and it was also noted that he had webbing of the neck and abnormal ears. His chromosome constitution was 46XY. Which of the following is the most probable diagnosis: congenital adrenal hyperplasia, Ullrich–Turner syndrome, Reifenstein's syndrome, testicular agenesis?

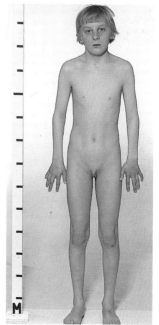

144

145

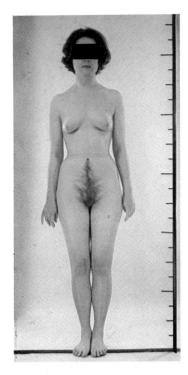

145 This patient presented with primary amenorrhoea and partial masculinisation. Investigation revealed an increase in plasma testosterone, a reduction in sex hormone binding globulin (SHBG) and raised urinary 17-oxosteroids with a normal female (46XX) chromosome constitution. Which of the following diagnoses fits these findings: ovarian dysgenesis, Cushing's syndrome, arrhenoblastoma, congenital adrenal hyperplasia?

146

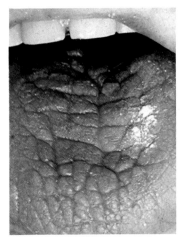

146 (a) Which diabetic complication might be associated with this appearance?
(b) Which of the following acute complications are seen in this condition:
    (i) reduced skin turgor,
    (ii) tachycardia and low-volume pulse,
    (iii) boils, carbuncles, or other infections,
    (iv) papilloedema,
    (v) acute neuropathy?

147 (a) What abnormality can be seen?

(b) Which of the following drugs may be responsible:

    (i) phenobarbitone,
    (ii) phenytoin,
    (iii) cortisol,
    (iv) prednisolone?

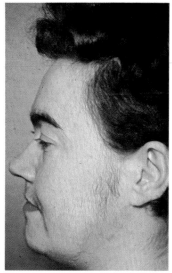

147

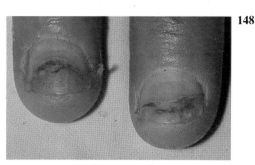

148

148 (a) This patient complained that she had had difficulty in keeping her finger nails clean. What condition does she exhibit?

(b) Which of the following statements about this condition are likely to be true?

    (i) It would be worth enquiring for symptoms of hyperthyroidism.
    (ii) A finding of pitting of the nails might help in the diagnosis.
    (iii) Iron deficiency could be a contributory factor.
    (iv) Such patients usually have associated localised myxoedema.
    (v) Beyond reassurance and treatment of the underlying condition, no local treatment to the nails is required.

149

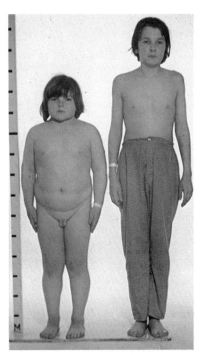

149 Two 13-year-old boys are shown. The child on the left is well below the third percentile for height. He was found to have a bone age of 9 years. No other significant symptoms were present. Which of the following endocrine conditions may be responsible: hypothyroidism, hypoadrenalism, hypoparathyroidism, diabetes mellitus?

150

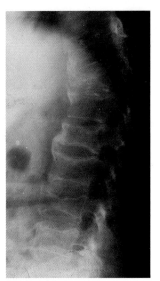

150 (a) What spinal abnormality is shown in this radiograph?
(b) Which of the following adrenal disorders may cause this abnormality:
    (i) congenital adrenal hyperplasia,
    (ii) Conn's syndrome,
    (iii) Addison's disease,
    (iv) ectopic ACTH syndrome,
    (v) Cushing's disease?

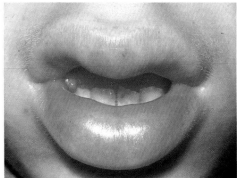
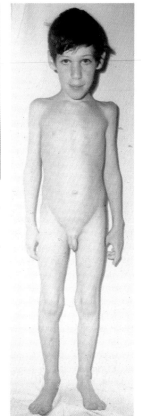

151, 152 (a) This 5-year-old boy was referred to hospital because of his unusual appearance. What is the likely diagnosis?
(b) Which of the following are features of this condition:
  (i) mucosal neuromas of the tongue,
  (ii) proximal myopathy,
  (iii) 'C cell' hyperplasia of the thyroid,
  (iv) phaeochromocytoma confined to one adrenal medulla,
  (v) insulin-secreting islet-cell tumours?

153 This X-ray of the wrist of a 12-year-old boy, with short limbs and a moderate degree of dwarfism, shows considerable irregularity and dysplasia of the epiphyses. He also complained of morning stiffness, some muscular weakness and joint pain and stiffness, although there was no obvious abnormality of the joints on physical examination. Which of the following diagnoses fit the clinical and radiological features: multiple epiphyseal dysplasia, osteogenesis imperfecta, rickets, hypoparathyroidism?

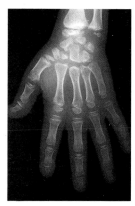

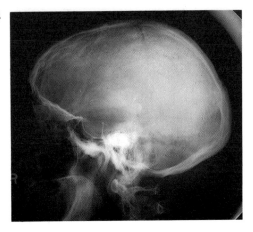

154 (a) This is the pituitary fossa of a 25-year-old man who attended casualty following a fall when he struck his head and became unconscious for 10 minutes. After taking the skull X-ray and observing the appearance of the pituitary fossa the patient was questioned about features of pituitary disease but was entirely asymptomatic. He was noted to have rather rugged features and moderately large hands and feet but was a manual worker. The skin on the back of his hands was thicker than normal. What is the abnormality shown and what diagnosis comes to mind?

(b) Which of the following statements about this condition are correct?

(i) It is often asymptomatic.

(ii) It may present with acroparaesthesiae.

(iii) Hypertension is common.

(iv) Suppression of growth hormone (GH) levels to < 5 mU/l during a glucose tolerance test excludes the diagnosis.

(v) The pituitary fossa is always enlarged in patients with acromegaly so a normal sized pituitary fossa excludes the diagnosis.

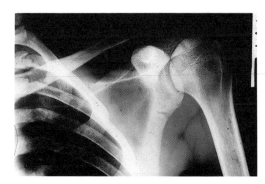

155 (a) What abnormality is shown on this X-ray?
(b) Which of the following symptoms are likely to be present in the patient: muscle weakness, bone tenderness, atrophy of the nails, hair loss?

156 This short, obese boy with poorly developed genitalia was found to have diabetes mellitus. Which of the following diagnoses fit the clinical picture: Cushing's syndrome, Noonan's (male Turner's) syndrome, Lawrence–Moon–Biedl syndrome, Prader–Willi syndrome?

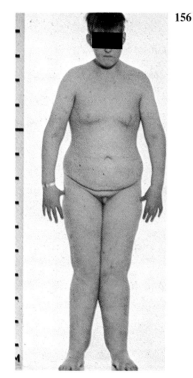

157

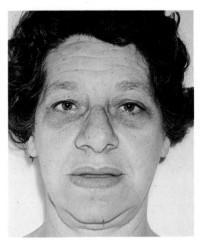

157 (a) This woman has an endocrine disorder which led to diabetes mellitus. What endocrine condition is it and is the associated diabetes frequently complicated by ketoacidosis?

(b) Which of the following endocrine conditions may be complicated by diabetes mellitus: Cushing's syndrome, acromegaly, non-secretory pituitary adenoma, glucagonoma, hyperthyroidism, aldosteronism?

158

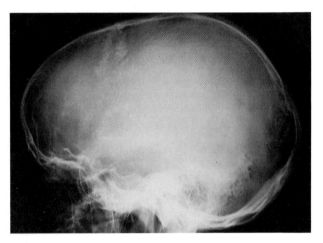

158 (a) This skull X-ray shows extensive intracranial calcification, particularly in the region of the basal ganglia. What is the likely cause?

(b) Which of the following may also be associated with this condition:
   (i) epilepsy,
   (ii) papilloedema,
   (iii) Parkinson's disease,
   (iv) deafness,
   (v) oculomotor palsy?

159 (a) This 50-year-old man complained of increasing prominence of the right eye of 2 months' duration. He was otherwise well and had no symptoms suggestive of thyroid disease. There had been some discomfort in the region of the eye. Which of the following statements is likely to be correct and why?

(i) He is likely to be suffering from the ophthalmic form of Graves' disease.

(ii) The appearance of his eyes is of help in establishing a diagnosis.

(b) With regard to his investigation: Which investigation would you do first? What additional investigation might well be helpful? Would operative intervention be likely to prove helpful?

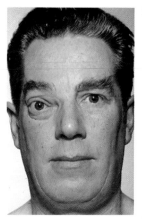

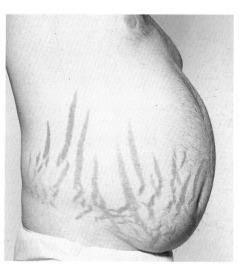

160 (a) What physical sign is shown in this photograph?

(b) With what syndrome is this characteristically associated?

(c) What other clinical condition may give rise to the same physical sign?

(d) What is the underlying cause of this skin abnormality?

(e) Is this sign restricted to women who have borne children?

161

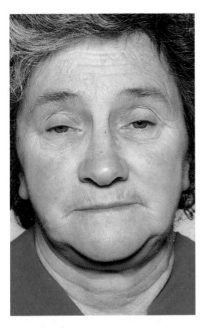

161 (a) What clinical condition may this 45-year-old woman be suffering from?

(b) Which of the following statements about this patient are likely to be true?

   (i) She could well be depressed.

   (ii) She exhibits bilateral ptosis.

   (iii) Myasthenia gravis should be excluded.

   (iv) A chest X-ray may well show evidence of a pericardial effusion.

   (v) She is likely to have circulating thyroid peroxidase antibodies.

162

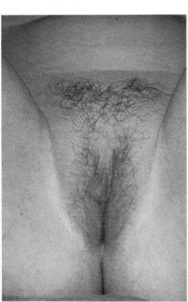

162 These immature external genitalia were found on examination in a 19-year-old woman with poorly developed secondary sexual characteristics and primary amenorrhoea whose chromosome constitution was found to be 46XX. Which of the following statements are likely to be true?

   (i) The uterus and fallopian tubes will be absent.

   (ii) Ovarian dysgenesis will be present.

   (iii) Primitive testicular tissue will be present.

   (iv) There is an increased risk of malignant gonadal tumours.

   (v) The patient will have a eunuchoid appearance.

163 (a) This 45-year-old woman complained of a swelling in the left side of the neck following a thyroidectomy for hyperthyroid Graves' disease 10 years previously. She was euthyroid and had a 5 cm diameter, smooth, firm, unattached nodule at the side of the swelling. What is the likely cause?

(b) Which of the following investigations might prove helpful in her case:
   (i) thyrotrophin-receptor antibody (TRAb) measurement,
   (ii) ultrasound of the neck,
   (iii) ^{123}I scan of the thyroid,
   (iv) serum calcium and phosphate levels,
   (v) fine-needle aspiration biopsy of the nodule?

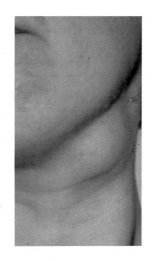

164 (a) The illustration shows a patient with spasmodic involuntary contractions of the carpal muscles. What is this physical sign?

(b) Which of the following metabolic abnormalities may be associated with this phenomenon: hypokalaemia, hypocalcaemia, hypoglycaemia, hypomagnesaemia?

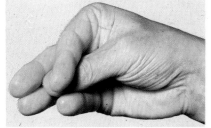

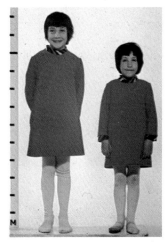

165 One of these 7½-year-old monozygotic twins shows severe growth retardation. The history revealed that there had been a major disparity in birth weight between the two. Which of the following fit the clinical picture: placental insufficiency, intrauterine infection, achondroplasia, maternal hypothyroidism?

166

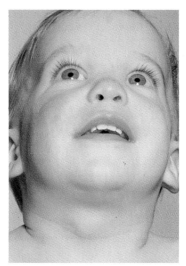

166 (a) This 4-year-old boy had a 2.5 cm smooth swelling in the midline of the neck above the thyroid cartilage, which moved upwards on swallowing. He was clinically euthyroid. What is the likely diagnosis?

(b) Which of the following statements about this condition are true?

(i) It represents a congenital defect in the descent of the thyroid from the base of the tongue.

(ii) Such patients have entirely normal thyroid function.

(iii) It is mandatory to confirm the presence of normal thyroid tissue by ultrasound or scanning before surgical removal of the lesion.

(iv) There is an increased risk of malignancy in such lesions.

(v) A decreased serum calcitonin level is found since the presence of the lesion signifies a defect in location of the ultimobranchial body.

167

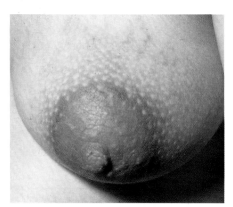

167 (a) What does this picture illustrate?

(b) Which of the following conditions could be associated with this appearance: racial origin, pregnancy, stilboestrol therapy, hyperthyroidism, Addison's disease?

168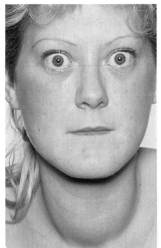

168 (a) This 30-year-old woman was clinically and biochemically hyperthyroid. What disease does she typify and what clinical features of this disease does she illustrate?

(b) Which of the following conditions are recognised causes of hyperthyroidism: amiodarone therapy, post-partum thyroiditis, bronchogenic carcinoma, choriocarcinoma, de Quervain's thyroiditis?

169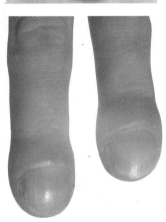

170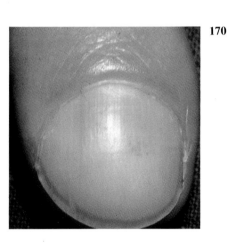

169, 170 (a) These are the hands of a 25-year-old woman with Graves' disease and hyperthyroidism. What do they illustrate?

(b) Which of the following statements are likely to be correct?
  (i) The changes are unlikely to be related to her Graves' disease.
  (ii) She is likely to exhibit evidence of localised myxoedema.
  (iii) She is likely to have eye signs of Graves' disease.
  (iv) Her nail signs will remit with treatment of her hyperthyroidism.
  (v) X-ray of her hands might help to distinguish the cause.

171

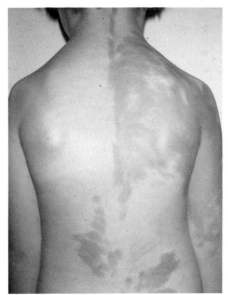

171 (a) This patient with precocious puberty was found to have the pigmentation illustrated. What is the probable diagnosis?
(b) Which of the following endocrine conditions may be associated with this condition: goitre, acromegaly, gynaecomastia, Cushing's syndrome?

172

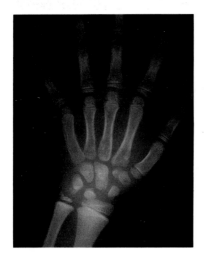

172 This X-ray is of the hand of a 4-year-old child, although the bone age is that of a 9-year-old. Which of the following conditions may be associated with this degree of advancement of bone age:
  (i) pinealoma,
  (ii) gigantism,
  (iii) congenital adrenal hyperplasia,
  (iv) Marfan's syndrome?

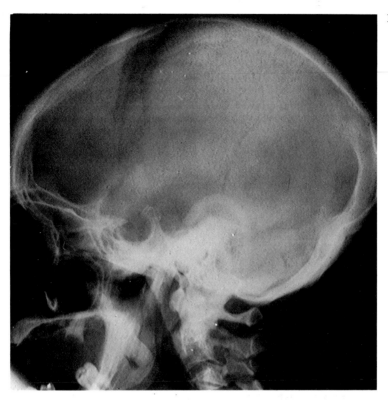

173 (a) This skull X-ray was from a 50-year-old woman who complained of bitemporal headaches of 6 months' duration. On examination she appeared to be mildly hypothyroid and had a mid-line neck swelling 4 cm in diameter, just below the thyroid cartilage. What does the skull X-ray show and what underlying condition do you suspect?
(b) Which of the following are recognised features of the condition:
    (i) visual field defects,
    (ii) serum thyroid-stimulating hormone (TSH) level of < 20 mU/l,
    (iii) shrinkage of the pituitary lesion with thyroxine,
    (iv) shortness of stature,
    (v) strongly positive thyroid peroxidase antibodies?

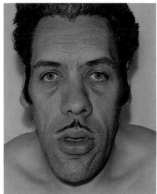

174 (a) What is the diagnosis?
(b) Which of the following statements about this condition are true?
  (i) It is usually due to eosinophilic (somatotroph) hyperplasia.
  (ii) It is rarely due to ectopic production of a growth hormone-releasing factor (GRF).
  (iii) It is a cause of macroglossia.
  (iv) A thick skin is an important physical sign in the diagnosis.
  (v) Galactorrhoea is a common sign.

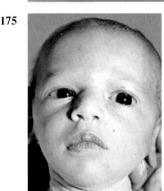

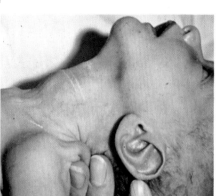

175, 176 This 5-day-old boy was losing weight. He had a pulse rate of 160/min with runs of atrial fibrillation and an apical Grade II pansystolic murmur. His mother had been treated with radioiodine for hyperthyroid Graves' disease 5 years previously and was maintained on thyroxine 0.15 mg daily for post-radioiodine hypothyroidism. Which of the following statements about this child are likely to be correct?
  (i) A goitre is likely to be present in the child.
  (ii) The mother is also likely to have a goitre.
  (iii) The child is in urgent need of investigation and treatment.
  (iv) The mother is likely to have high levels of thyrotrophin receptor antibodies (TRAb).
  (v) The child's underlying condition is likely to remit spontaneously in a few months' time.

177 (a) This 30-year-old man complained of tall stature (2.09 m), lack of energy, and difficulty in having a sexual relationship. What is the likely diagnosis?
(b) What clinical features does he exhibit and what investigations would you consider relevant to establish the primary diagnosis?

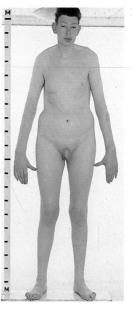

178 (a) This chest X-ray was taken from a 40-year-old patient with long-standing acromegaly, who complained of shortness of breath on exertion and swelling of the ankles. The patient was normotensive with mild congestive cardiac failure and cardiomegaly. There was clinical evidence of acromegaly. What abnormality is shown on the X-ray, and what was the sex of the patient?
(b) Which of the following might have contributed to the abnormality shown on the X-ray: hypertension, ischaemic heart disease, pericardial effusion, cardiomyopathy, amyloidosis?

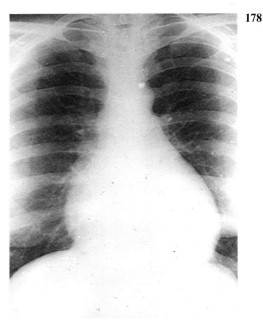

179

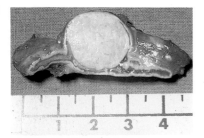

179 This is the cut surface of an adenoma of the adrenal zona glomerulosa, showing the characteristic yellow colour of the lesion.
(a) What syndrome is associated with this tumour?
(b) Which of the following clinical features are likely to be present: hypertension, muscle weakness, tetany, loss of pubic and axillary hair, oedema?

180

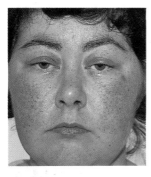

180 (a) What is the probable diagnosis in this woman?
(b) Which of the following symptoms are likely to be present: depression, amenorrhoea, tinnitus, bronchospasm, diarrhoea?

181

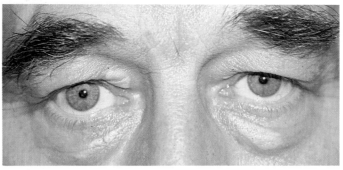

181 (a) What condition is illustrated?
(b) Which of the following statements about this condition are true?

(i) The serum cholesterol and triglycerides are often normal in affected patients.
(ii) The condition is common in hyperthyroidism.
(iii) It may be associated with a familial hyperlipidaemia.
(iv) Vigorous cholesterol-lowering therapy may lead to its resolution.
(v) It may be associated with diabetes mellitus.

182 (a) What is the likely diagnosis of this 10-year-old girl, who had stopped growing in height 2 years previously?
(b) Which of the following are recognised features of this condition: galactorrhoea, skin pigmentation, precocious puberty, nephrocalcinosis, epilepsy.

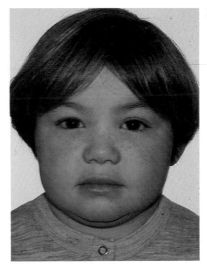

182

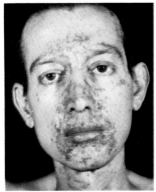

83

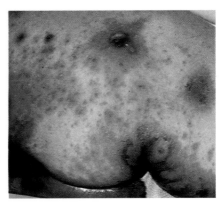

184

183, 184 (a) What endocrine condition is illustrated here?
(b) Which of the following statements about this condition are true?
   (i) Glossitis is frequently present.
   (ii) The rash cannot be induced by the administration of glucagon.
   (iii) Thrombo-embolism is a known complication.
   (iv) Amelioration of the rash can be induced by therapy with magnesium.
   (v) The patients are usually severely diabetic with ketoacidosis.

185

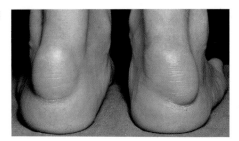

186

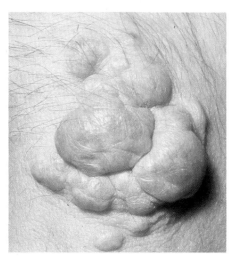

187

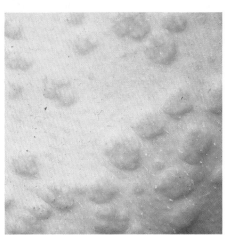

185–187 (a) These skin lesions were observed in a woman with poorly controlled insulin-dependent diabetes mellitus. What are they?

(b) Which of these statements about this condition are true?

(i) The serum cholesterol is raised.

(ii) Triglyceride levels are normal.

(iii) Low-density lipoprotein (LDL)–cholesterol levels remain normal.

(iv) On standing, the serum may appear milky.

(v) Eruptive xanthomas persist despite good control of the diabetes.

188 This female patient presented with secondary amenorrhoea, frontal baldness, deepening of the voice and breast atrophy. Investigations showed an increase in testosterone, reduced sex hormone binding globulin (SHBG) levels and normal urinary 17-oxogenic and oxosteroids. Which of the following diagnoses fit the clinical picture:
  (i) androgen administration,
  (ii) Cushing's syndrome,
  (iii) congenital adrenal hyperplasia,
  (iv) virilising adrenal adenoma,
  (v) arrhenoblastoma?

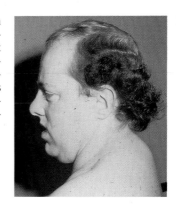

189 This patient, who had received no medication, presented with primary amenorrhoea and was found on investigation to be chromatin negative on buccal smear and to have a 46XY karyotype. Which of the following diagnoses fits these findings: Turner's syndrome, Ullrich–Turner syndrome, congenital adrenal hyperplasia, testicular feminisation?

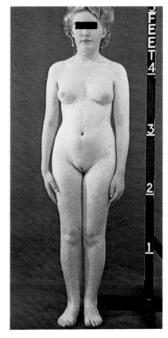

190

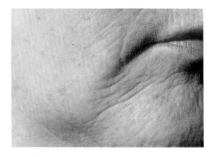

190 (a) What lesion is shown and what does it imply?
(b) Which of the following clinical and laboratory features might confirm a pituitary cause:
  (i) fine wrinkling of the skin,
  (ii) thin skin, shown by picking up a fold of skin on the back of the patient's hand,
  (iii) loss of hair,
  (iv) low free testosterone,
  (v) elevation of FSH with low LH?

191

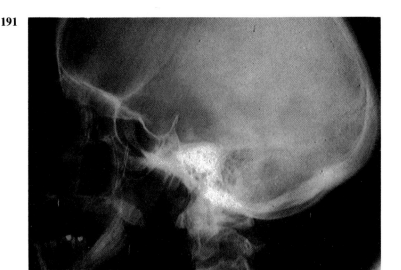

191 (a) This skull X-ray was obtained from an 18-year-old boy who complained of short stature and recent thirst and headaches. What does the X-ray show?
(b) Which of the following problems may be associated with this condition: diabetes insipidus, hyperphagia, loss of short-term memory, somnolence, hypothermia?

192 This young man, with abnormal tallness of stature, was noted to have obvious prognathism, a high-arched palate and a range of neuromuscular problems including ataxia, mental retardation and abnormal clumsiness. His growth hormone secretion was normal. Which of the following fit the clinical picture: Marfan's syndrome, XYY syndrome, Kallmann's syndrome, Soto's syndrome?

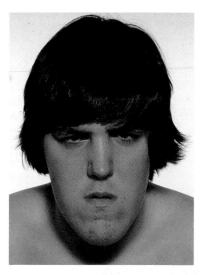

193 This middle-aged woman presented with severe and increasing pigmentation and the passage of dark urine. Which of the following investigations might contribute to identifying the underlying cause:

(i) chest X-ray,
(ii) serum calcium,
(iii) glucose tolerance test,
(iv) plasma ACTH,
(v) plasma growth hormone?

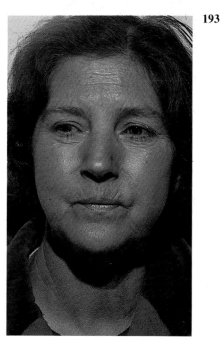

194

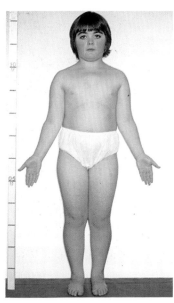

194 (a) This girl was brought to the clinic on account of shortness of stature and delayed puberty. What physical sign is shown which suggested the diagnosis?

(b) Which of the following features may be associated with this syndrome:

  (i) coarctation of the aorta,
  (ii) hypothyroidism,
  (iii) horseshoe kidney,
  (iv) polycystic kidneys,
  (v) dextrocardia?

195

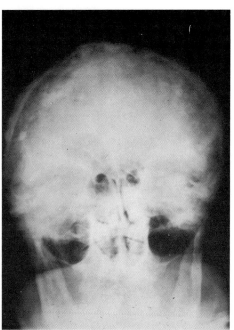

195 (a) Describe the radiological abnormalities shown.

(b) Which of the following biochemical findings are likely in this condition: raised serum parathyroid hormone, raised serum IgG, raised alkaline phosphatase, raised phosphate?

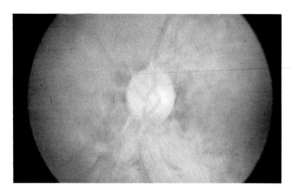

196 (a) This fundal photograph was from a young woman who had recently developed insulin-dependent diabetes mellitus (IDDM). What abnormality does it show?

(b) Which of the following statements about IDDM are true?

    (i) Endogenous insulin secretion cannot be estimated by measuring circulating C-peptide concentrations.

    (ii) The majority of patients with IDDM present before the age of 30.

    (iii) Patients presenting with IDDM do not usually have ketonuria.

    (iv) More than 90% of the B-cell mass must be destroyed before clinical diabetes appears.

    (v) IDDM is associated with the HLA antigens DR2 and DR4.

197 (a) This patient complained that her nails had become hardened, grooved and discoloured and that the ends were breaking. What is the probable diagnosis?

(b) Which of the following endocrine/metabolic conditions may predispose to this disorder:

    (i) hyperthyroidism,
    (ii) diabetes mellitus,
    (iii) Turner's syndrome,
    (iv) hypoparathyroidism?

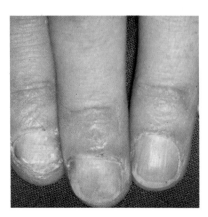

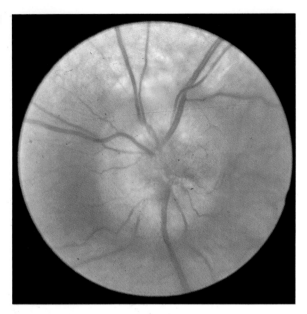

198 (a) What is wrong with this fundus?

(b) Which of the following statements about the optic nerve and optic pathways are correct?

(i) The condition is common in patients with a pituitary tumour.

(ii) In the presence of a pituitary tumour the condition would indicate suprasellar extension.

(iii) Suprasellar extension of a pituitary tumour always causes bitemporal hemianopia.

(iv) Suprasellar extension of a pituitary tumour can occur without any defect in the visual fields.

(v) The condition may progress to optic atrophy even after the causative suprasellar extension has been removed.

199 (a) This middle-aged woman with severe shortness of stature, gave a history of repeated fractures throughout her life, leading to considerable deformities of the limbs. What is the probable diagnosis?

(b) Which of the following statements are true?

(i) Inheritance is as an autosomal dominant.

(ii) Inheritance is as an autosomal recessive.

(iii) Blindness may be associated with the condition.

(iv) Deafness may be associated with the condition.

(v) Dental abnormalities may be associated with this disorder.

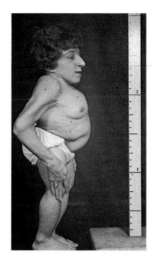

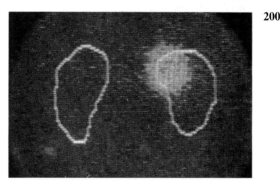

200 The MIBG (metaiodobenzylguanidine) scan shows a phaeochromocytoma. Which of the following statements are true of phaeochromocytoma?

(i) The tumours are always benign.

(ii) The tumours may be found in sympathetic tissue outside the adrenal medulla.

(iii) Phaeochromocytoma accounts for 5% of all cases of hypertension.

(iv) Paroxysmal hypertension is characteristic.

(v) A fall in blood pressure with phentolamine is diagnostic of phaeochromocytoma.

201

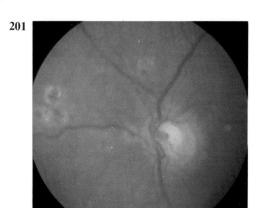

202

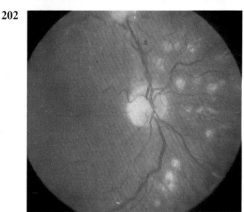

203

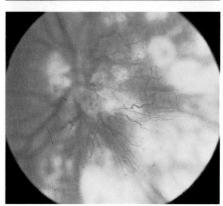

201–203 (a) What condition is illustrated in these retinal photographs?

(b) Which of the following statements about this procedure are correct?

(i) It helps to prevent progression of certain types of diabetic retinopathy.

(ii) Pain may be experienced by the patient during the procedure.

(iii) It produces a retinal picture which is often mistaken for retinitis pigmentosa.

(iv) It should be avoided in insulin-dependent diabetics.

204 This patient has Cushing's syndrome. Which of the following statements about this syndrome are correct?

(i) The most common cause of Cushing's syndrome is the administration of steroids or ACTH.

(ii) The most common cause of spontaneously occurring Cushing's syndrome (i.e. not related to steroid or ACTH administration) is an adrenal adenoma.

(iii) Pigmentation is a common feature of adrenal adenoma.

(iv) Cushing's disease describes Cushing's syndrome of hypothalamic–pituitary origin.

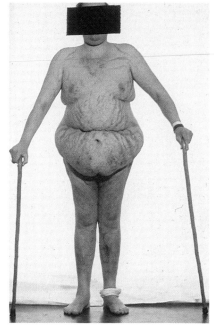

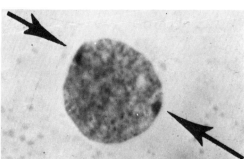

205 (a) This cell is from a buccal smear. What cellular feature is highlighted by the two arrows?
(b) Which of the following conditions may be associated with this abnormality:
  (i) Turner's syndrome,
  (ii) Ullrich–Turner syndrome,
  (iii) Klinefelter's syndrome,
  (iv) XXXY disorder?

206

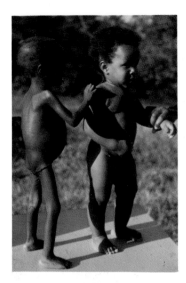

206 (a) The 3½-year-old child on the left is shown compared with a healthy child of 10 months. What is the probable diagnosis?

(b) Which of the following metabolic abnormalities may be associated with this condition: hyperglycaemia, hypoalbuminaemia, raised blood urea, hypercholesterolaemia?

207

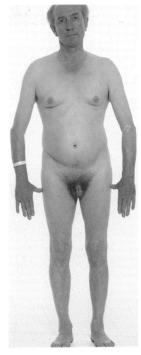

207 (a) This 50-year-old man presented with a 6-month history of painful bilateral gynaecomastia. His skin showed some purple striae over the buttocks and there was a ballottable 10 cm mass palpable in the left hypochondrium. What is the likely diagnosis?

(b) Which of the following statements about this condition are likely to be true?

(i) The gynaecomastia will be due to cortisol secretion from the lesion.

(ii) Such lesions commonly secrete a variety of adrenocortical hormones.

(iii) The cortisol secretion rate may well be elevated.

(iv) Measurement of 24-hour urinary oxosteroids may be helpful in the diagnosis.

(v) The prognosis for 5-year survival will be good.

(vi) The lesion should be easily demonstrated by ultrasound examination.

208 (a) What abnormality is shown in this X-ray?
(b) Which of the following conditions is likely to be responsible: primary hyperparathyroidism, secondary hyperparathyroidism, Paget's disease, osteomalacia?

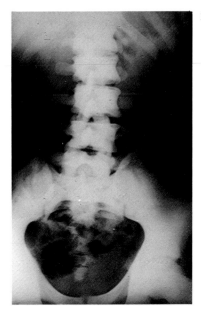

209 (a) What physical sign is shown in this 32-year-old woman?
(b) Which of the following conditions may be responsible:
  (i) pituitary failure,
  (ii) hyperthyroidism,
  (iii) Turner's syndrome,
  (iv) acromegaly,
  (v) Addison's disease?

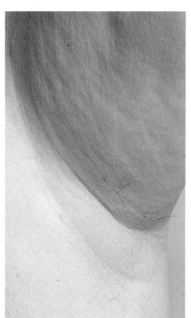

210

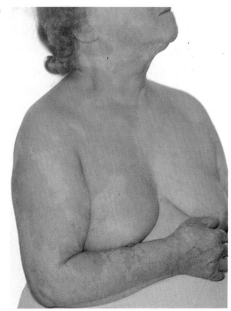

210, 211 (a) This woman was noted to have unilateral pigmentation of the neck which had been present from birth. What is the likely diagnosis?

(b) List the endocrine disorders which go along with this condition.

211

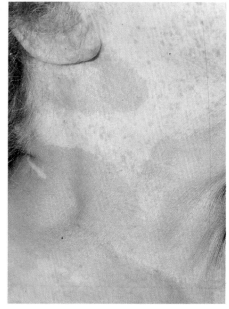

212 These boys are both 14 years old. Which of the following conditions may be responsible for the retardation of growth in the one on the left: bronchiectasis, cystic fibrosis, intestinal malabsorption, emotional deprivation, congenital heart disease?

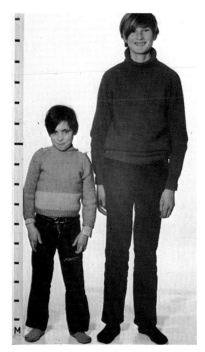

213 (a) What chronic complication of diabetes mellitus is illustrated here?
(b) Which of the following are seen in the chronic neuropathy of diabetes mellitus?

   (i) A sensory neuropathy causing trophic ulceration.
   (ii) A Charcot joint.
   (iii) A motor neuropathy causing proximal muscle weakness and wasting.
   (iv) Mononeuritis multiplex.
   (v) Autonomic neuropathy causing diarrhoea.

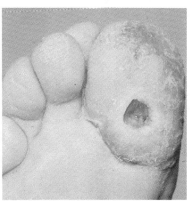

214

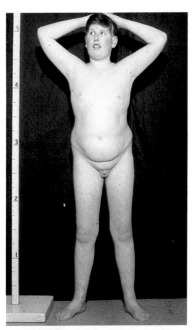

214 This blind 21-year-old has failed to develop pubertal changes. Which of the following diagnoses fit the clinical picture: craniopharyngioma, Klinefelter's syndrome, XYY syndrome, Ullrich–Turner syndrome?

215

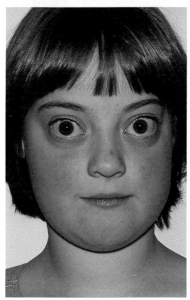

215 (a) What is the likely diagnosis in this 9-year-old girl who was brought to the endocrine clinic having lost 4 kg in weight over a 3-month period while having a voracious appetite?

(b) Which of the following statements about this condition are true?

(i) It occurs as commonly in children as in adults.

(ii) It has a tendency to relapse after drug treatment.

(iii) There is commonly a family history of autoimmune disease.

(iv) It is likely that circulating TPO (thyroid peroxidase) antibodies will be present.

(v) It may be associated with accelerated linear growth.

ANSWERS

1 (i), (ii), (iii) and (v) are true. The possibility of previous torsion of the testes and of mumps orchitis should be excluded. In this case, enquiry about the patient's sense of smell revealed the diagnosis. He suffers from Kallmann's syndrome of hypogonadotrophic hypogonadism associated with anosmia. This is a familial condition which can occur in either sex but is more common in males. It is due to a deficiency in production of gonadotrophin-releasing hormone.

2 (a) The X-ray shows a bronchial carcinoma.
(b) Cushing's syndrome, hypercalcaemia or Addison's disease. Cushing's syndrome may result from the secretion of ACTH by a malignant neoplasm—most commonly an oat cell carcinoma or bronchial carcinoid. Hypercalcaemia may be associated with a bronchial carcinoma (usually a squamous cell tumour) without bony metastases. This almost always results from the secretion of an ectopic parathyroid hormone related protein. Addison's disease rarely results from infiltration and destruction of both adrenal cortices by secondary deposits from a bronchial carcinoma.

3 (a) Wasting of the thenar eminence due to median nerve damage usually due to compression of the nerve at the wrist in the carpal tunnel syndrome.
(b) Statements (ii) and (v) are true. The syndrome is most common in middle-aged women and usually no underlying cause can be found. It is a common presenting symptom in acromegaly due to an increase in bone and soft tissue in the region of the carpal tunnel. Medical treatment with local corticosteroid injections, splinting and reduced use may suffice in mild cases. Nerve conduction studies can be helpful in confirming the diagnosis. Symptoms are always worse in bed at night and often eased by hanging the arms down over the edge of the bed.

4 (a) Hirsutism.
(b) Hirsutism is a known complication of therapy with all of these drugs except for paracetamol.

5, 6 (a) The Laurence–Moon–Biedl syndrome.
(b) The clinical features illustrated are: obesity, hypogonadism, and polydactyly. The hypothalamus is the site of the lesion.

7 (a) Congestive ophthalmopathy. This term is preferred to malignant exophthalmos since exophthalmos may not be present.
(b) Statements (i) and (v) are correct. There is a major risk to vision if prompt, effective treatment is not initiated. Papilloedema is not invariable even in the presence of clear optic nerve compression. Macular oedema is common and defects in red–green colour vision confirm optic nerve compression.

8 (a) The man has acromegaly, his sister may have had a parathyroidectomy for hyperparathyroidism causing her renal calculi. The presence of two separate endocrine disorders in first degree relatives affecting the pituitary and parathyroid glands makes it important to consider the diagnosis of multiple endocrine neoplasia Type I (MEN I).
(b) Disorders (i), (ii), (iii), (v) and (vi) are associated with this condition. Tumours of the pituitary, parathyroid, pancreas and adrenal are seen in MEN I. Medullary carcinoma of the thyroid and phaeochromocytomas are seen in MEN II.

9 These patients have characteristics (i) and (v)—they are also of above average height and occasionally hypogonadal.

10, 11 (a) She shows unilateral exophthalmos due to the ophthalmic form of Graves' disease. This is defined as the eye signs of Graves' disease in a patient who is clinically and biochemically not hyperthyroid and gives no past history of hyperthyroidism.

(b) The CT scan shows enlargement of the medial and lateral recti on the affected side and no evidence of an orbital tumour. It supports a diagnosis of Graves' ophthalmopathy.

12 (a) Cushing's syndrome.

(b) Investigations (iv) and (v) are essential. The most valuable tests to estab-' lish a diagnosis of Cushing's syndrome are measurement of the urinary free cortisol and the measurement of the circadian rhythm of cortisol. It is essential for the latter investigation to include a midnight sample and to ensure that the patient does not know that a sample is to be taken and is asleep immediately before venesection since cortisol is a stress hormone. Presence of a circadian rhythm excludes the diagnosis. Elevation of serum sodium is variable and non-specific; morning plasma cortisol alone may be elevated by stress and may not be significantly raised above normal levels in Cushing's syndrome and plasma ACTH is only raised in Cushing's syndrome of hypothalamic-pituitary origin or in the ectopic ACTH syndrome.

13 The likely diagnosis is pulmonary tuberculosis which is more common in diabetics. The chest X-ray shows tuberculous consolidation and cavities at the right apex and a left sided pleural effusion.

14 Hyperparathyroidism. The X-ray shows the characteristic granular or mottled appearance (often described as ground glass) which may include some cystic areas. Deposits of myeloma or secondary carcinoma typically show clear lytic areas (the intervening bone being normal) and in Paget's disease the bones are expanded and deformed with loss of corticomedullary definition and a coarse trabecular pattern.

15 (a) The scan shows a hypodense microadenoma compatible, with this history, with a prolactinoma.

(b) Statements (i), (iii) and (iv) are correct. Prolactinomas are usually hypodense on CT scanning after contrast. There is no convincing evidence that they result from oral contraceptive medication in man though prolactinomas can be induced by oestrogens in rats. Expansion of known prolactinomas can be induced by oestrogen injections. Microprolactinomas are much more common than macroprolactinomas except in selected cases presenting to a neurosurgeon. A modest elevation of prolactin, e.g. 1000 mU/l in a patient with a large tumour, suggests the possibility of a functional pituitary stalk section viz. a pseudo-prolactinoma. Most prolactinomas are radiosensitive.

16 (a) Sipple's syndrome of multiple endocrine neoplasia Type IIb (MEN IIb) in which medullary carcinoma of the thyroid may be associated with a marfanoid habitus and phaeochromocytomas and parathyroid adenomas.

(b) Statements (i), (ii), (iv) and (v) are true. Peripheral neuropathy is not a feature of MEN IIb. Such patients have a characteristic appearance and a marfanoid habitus.

17 (a) Haemochromatosis indicated by her pigmented appearance due to melanin and also iron deposition in the skin.

(b) All of these pancreatic conditions may lead to diabetes mellitus but in (iii) and (v) the diabetes is usually transient.

18–20 (a) He has a proximal myopathy and can only rise from a squatting position with difficulty.

(b) Proximal muscle weakness may be seen in Cushing's syndrome and diabetes mellitus. Severe proximal muscle weakness is very common in Cushing's syndrome and largely results from the increase in protein catabolism. Proximal muscle weakness results from an acute radiculopathy and is commonly seen in uncontrolled insulin-dependent diabetics or may follow a period of poor diabetic control. Muscle weakness is common in acromegaly and in Conn's syndrome but is not limited to the proximal muscle groups; generalised aches and pains are common is hypothyroidism and stiffness may be apparent—the muscles are increased in bulk in Hoffmann's syndrome.

21 (a) Cushing's syndrome commonly causes muscle weakness and excessive bruising due to the catabolic effects of the high cortisol levels.
(b) Investigations (i), (iii) and (v) would be appropriate. The best investigation to confirm excessive cortisol production is the 24-hour urinary free cortisol. The best time to estimate ACTH levels is 0900. In the presence of Cushing's syndrome of pituitary origin (Cushing's disease) or the ectopic ACTH syndrome, the plasma ACTH level will be raised; whereas with adrenal causes of Cushing's syndrome (i.e. an adrenal adenoma or carcinoma), the ACTH level will be suppressed. A chest X-ray might reveal a bronchial adenoma or carcinoma responsible for the ectopic ACTH syndrome. Plasma electrolytes may show a low potassium if the cortisol overproduction is severe.

22 Shortness of stature can result from any severe systemic illness. The features listed are characteristic of chronic renal failure. A low calcium and raised phosphate are also seen in association with growth retardation in hypoparathyroidism, but the blood urea level will be normal; both calcium and phosphate levels are low in rickets and the serum calcium is raised in vitamin D intoxication.

23 (a) A diabetic cataract.
(b) Statements (i), (iii) and (v) are correct. Diabetic cataracts can occur in young patients and are usually bilateral. They are associated with poor metabolic control. Senile cataracts occur more frequently and at an earlier age in diabetes. Diabetic cataracts typically have a snowflake appearance and occur in the subcapsular region of the lens.

24 (a) Autoimmune thyroid disease. All of the patients shown had significant titres of thyroid peroxidase antibodies.
(b) Conditions (i), (ii), (iii) and (iv) are known to be associated with autoimmune thyroid disease and fit into the category of organ-specific autoimmune disorders.

25, 26 (a) This hypothyroid woman had a pericardial effusion which resolved by the time of the second chest X-ray with thyroxine therapy.
(b) Body cavity effusions known to complicate hypothyroidism include ascites, uveal effusions visible on fundoscopy which impair vision, hydroceles and middle and inner ear effusions which contribute to the deafness, dizziness and occasionally true vertigo seen in hypothyroidism.

27 (i), (ii), (iii) and (v) are exhibited. Sclera is visible between the cornea and the upper lid indicating the presence of lid retraction. Sclera is also visible between the cornea and the lower lid indicating the presence of exophthalmos. There is some periorbital swelling affecting the upper lids. There is no evidence of ophthalmoplegia in the position of forward gaze though this would only be excluded by testing full eye movements. Conjunctival injection is clearly seen.

28 (a) The patient has obvious expansion of the skull characteristic of Paget's disease, leading to compression of the seventh cranial nerve and a facial palsy.
(b) (i) and (iv) may complicate the disease. Paget's disease may also cause lesions of other nerves which may be compressed in bony canals. The patient illustrated also has a hearing aid.

29, 30 (a) The Prader–Willi syndrome.
(b) Features (i) and (v) are seen. The obesity is due to hyperphagia of hypothalamic origin. The condition is often complicated by diabetes mellitus. Affected individuals are hypogonadal and have small hands and feet.

31–35 The correct match is:
31 Lipoatrophy.
32 Acromegaly.
33 Normal variant.
34 Hashimoto's disease and hypothyroidism.
35 Acromegaly.

36 (a) Shortening of the third, fourth and fifth metacarpals in a patient with pseudohypoparathyroidism.
(b) Tetany occurs due to hypocalcaemia, and exostoses (together with other skeletal and dental abnormalities) are common. Webbing of the neck is most frequently seen in Turner's syndrome. There is some overlap between the skeletal abnormalities of these two conditions, but characteristically there is only shortening of the fourth metacarpal in Turner's syndrome.

37 (a) The lateral skull X-ray shows a double floor of the pituitary fossa indicating asymmetrical expansion of a pituitary tumour.
(b) Investigations (i) and (ii) would be relevant. The most likely cause is a prolactinoma, the most common form of pituitary tumour. The diagnosis can be confirmed or refuted by measurement of the serum prolactin. Many such patients do not have galactorrhoea either spontaneously or on expression. Visual field examination is mandatory in all patients with pituitary tumours. Ultrasound examination of the ovaries, chest X-ray and karyotype are all irrelevant in this patient. A chromosomal anomaly causing infertility is most unlikely in a patient with a normal menstrual cycle.

38 (a) The voltage is low.
(b) Conditions (ii) and (iii) may be associated. This is a non-specific abnormality and cannot be relied upon for diagnostic purposes. These changes are generally reversed by treatment. A low-voltage ECG may also be seen in some non-endocrine disorders (e.g. pericardial effusion and some cardiomyopathies). The ECG in Conn's syndrome characteristically shows the changes of hypokalaemia with ST–T depression, U waves and ventricular premature contractions. There are no characteristic ECG changes in hypoparathyroidism.

39 (a) Shortening of the fourth metacarpal.
(b) This is a common skeletal abnormality in Turner's syndrome, which can be demonstrated clinically by asking the patient to clench a fist thus revealing the shortened metacarpal.

40 (a) Graves' disease with lid retraction and a goitre causing hyperthyroidism.
(b) Statements (ii), (iv) and (v) are correct. Occasionally, patients with hyperthyroidism gain weight if the increase in appetite more than compensates for the hypermetabolism. Thirst is common in hyperthyroidism though rarely complained of spontaneously. Increased appetite with loss of weight is also seen in diabetes mellitus and intestinal parasitic infections.

41, 42 Ptosis, lateral strabismus and a dilated right pupil. They imply a lesion of the third right cranial nerve due to lateral extension of a pituitary tumour into the cavernous sinus.

43 These findings are characteristic of progeria.

44 (a) Pendred's syndrome, a dyshormonogenetic goitre associated with nerve deafness due to a defect in the organification of iodine.
(b) Features (i), (ii), (iii) and (v) are recognised. The condition, like most examples of thyroid dyshormonogenesis, is inherited on an autosomal recessive basis. A positive perchlorate discharge test, where more than 10% of a dose of radioiodine is discharged from the thyroid after administration of 600 mg of potassium perchlorate by mouth, is diagnostic. Such goitres always recur after thyroidectomy unless full thyroxine therapy is instituted. The circulating level of MIT is normal. Because of decreased thyroid hormone formation and intrathyroidal iodine deficiency, the biochemical changes stated occur in this condition.

45 (a) Gyral calcification characteristic of the Sturge–Weber syndrome.
(b) Facial or intracranial haemangiomas are characteristic of this neuro-ectodermal syndrome. Phaeochromocytoma may be associated with any of this group of disorders.

46 (i), (ii) and (v) fit the picture. All these conditions may be associated with abnormal height. The majority of cases result from familial tallness of stature (the patient illustrated is an example). Patients with Klinefelter's syndrome are tall with eunuchoid proportions but also have poorly developed secondary sexual characteristics. Patients with congenital adrenal hyperplasia show accelerated growth prior to puberty but the epiphyses close early and the final height is reduced.

47 (a) Acanthosis nigricans.
(b) Statements (i) and (iii) are true. The condition is not related to malignant melanoma. It may be associated with other malignancies. It does not resolve spontaneously.

48 The child had severe hypothyroidism with a delay in growth and skeletal maturation. Cushing's syndrome also retards linear growth and delays skeletal maturation.

49–53 The correct match is:
49 Furunculosis.
50 Acanthosis nigricans.
51 Diabetic dermopathy.
52 Necrobiosis lipoidica.
53 Granuloma annulare.

54 (a) Galactorrhoea. The PRL level should be elevated.
(b) Statements (i), (iii), (iv) and (v) are true. Galactorrhoea and gynaecomastia are separate signs with different causes. Galactorrhoea is usually not accompanied by gynaecomastia. Gynaecomastia is best detected by pressure with the flat hand against the chest wall. It is usually due to oestrogen/androgen imbalance with excess oestrogen levels. Increased oestrogen ingestion can lead to increased PRL production in man, and in certain animals to the development of a prolactinoma. Quite often patients with hyper-prolactinaemia do not exhibit galactorrhoea.

55 (a) Klinefelter's syndrome. The majority of patients have an XXY chromosome constitution but occasionally other abnormalities—XY/XXY mosaics, XXYY, XXXY, XXXXY and XXXYY may be seen. Pituitary function is normal and the increase in height is due to delayed epiphyseal closure resulting from the hypogonadism.

(b) Statements (i) and (ii) are true. Patients with Klinefelter's syndrome have seminiferous tubule dysgenesis with low testosterone levels and high gonadotrophins resulting from lack of feedback inhibition.

56 (a) Hypertrichosis lanuginosa. The patient has an excess of soft, downy or vellus hair.

(b) This condition is associated with malignant neoplasms, most commonly carcinoma of the bronchus. An increase in downy hair may also be seen in anorexia nervosa but it does not become as luxuriant as that illustrated.

57 This association is characteristic of Kallmann's syndrome. The other syndromes are not associated with anosmia and the patient does not show the somatic features of Turner's syndrome. Congenital adrenal hyperplasia in the female is also associated with virilism.

58 (a) Galactorrhoea, defined as inappropriate milk secretion from the breast.

(b) Investigations (ii), (iv) and (v) would help in identification. A low serum thyroxine indicating hypothyroidism is a known cause of galactorrhoea. A lateral skull X-ray may reveal the presence of an enlarged pituitary fossa or show evidence of a pituitary or hypothalamic lesion. A random plasma cortisol if low supports a diagnosis of secondary hypoadrenalism but if normal does not rule out partial adrenocorticotrophin (ACTH) deficiency.

59 (a) Vitiligo.

(b) Statements (i), (ii), (iii) and (v) are correct. Some depigmentation of the skin may have been present from birth. Vitiligo is an 'almost-symmetrical' condition and there is likely to be some depigmentation in the other axilla. Vitiligo is associated with the organ-specific autoimmune diseases such as Hashimoto's disease, pernicious anaemia and Addison's disease. Vitiligo is associated with leucotrichia-depigmentation of the hair. Vitiligo is usually surrounded by an area of increased pigmentation.

60 (a) A thyroid neoplasm.

(b) Features (ii), (iii), (iv) and (v) would suggest malignancy. Although asymmetry is a feature of thyroid malignancy, many nodular goitres are asymmetrical and this finding alone is not highly suspicious of malignancy. Rapid, painful increase in size can also be seen due to haemorrhage into a thyroid nodule but in this case the swelling and discomfort resolve within a few weeks.

61 (a) Lipoatrophic diabetes.

(b) All of the clinical features listed may be associated with this rare form of diabetes.

62 (a) Fine needle aspiration biopsy of the thyroid.

(b) Statements (i), (ii) and (iii) are correct. It is now a standard diagnostic test for all patients with thyroid nodules. It is not possible to distinguish follicular adenomas from carcinomas by this technique, all follicular lesions require subsequent surgical exploration and excision. It is most helpful in diagnosing thyroid cysts, in aspirating them and in obtaining cyst fluid for cytology. It does not clearly separate all malignant from benign thyroid lesions. It is generally relatively pain-free and does not require either a local anaesthetic or sedation.

63–65 (a) **63** Insulin hypertrophy. **64** Insulin atrophy. **65** Insulin fibrosis.

(b) The complications of insulin therapy may improve spontaneously and can be avoided and treated by the use of neutral, highly purified insulin and by its injection into an affected area. Insulin fibrosis results from over-frequent injection at a single or limited number of sites and can lead to variability in the rate of insulin absorption.

66 (a) The pyelogram shows loss of the renal cortex and clubbing of the calyces suggesting chronic pyelonephritis.
(b) Complications (i) to (iv) may be seen. Hypertension is a common complication of diabetic renal disease. Severe infection can lead to a necrotising papillitis. Diabetic glomerulosclerosis—the Kimmelstiel–Wilson syndrome—may progress to renal failure and is a cause of the nephrotic syndrome.

67 (a) Widening and cupping of the epiphyseal plates in a child due to rickets.
(b) Calcium and phosphate levels are both reduced in rickets. Serum alkaline phosphatase and urinary hydroxyproline are both elevated reflecting the increased turnover of bone.

68, 69 (a) Superior mediastinal obstruction.
(b) This patient had a retro-sternal goitre with superior vena caval obstruction revealed on the venogram (**69**). Oesophageal and tracheal compression were indicated by the dysphagia and stridor. A similar syndrome can be produced by a bronchogenic carcinoma or by a mediastinal lymphoma and histological confirmation may be required by fine needle biopsy.

70 (a) Diabetes mellitus secondary to Cushing's syndrome.
(b) Statements (i) and (ii) are correct. Polyuria and nocturia may result from the effects of cortisol on the circadian rhythm of water and electrolyte excretion. Cortisol impairs peripheral glucose utilisation. Carbohydrate tolerance is impaired in 30–70% of patients with Cushing's syndrome and is almost always abnormal in the ectopic ACTH syndrome. The diabetes associated with Cushing's syndrome may not be easily controlled and may require insulin therapy.

71 (a) Klinefelter's syndrome.
(b) Statements (i), (ii), (iii) and (v) are true. Klinefelter's syndrome usually results from a 47XXY karyotype but other karyotypes e.g., 48XXYY, 48XXXY, 46XY/47XXY mosaicism or rarely 46XX may occur. The Leydig cells appear either normal or hyperplastic. Plasma testosterone levels may fall within the normal range and the severity of the hypogonadism is variable. The serum FSH is invariably raised and the LH usually elevated. One must exercise care in giving testosterone to such patients who may be immature in their behaviour and can become violent in response to androgens.

72 (a) Shortness of stature due to hypopituitarism, primary thyroid failure or Turner's syndrome.
(b) Short stature, immature facies, immature breasts with pigmented (Dodd's) nipples due to stilboestrol therapy and lack of pubic hair. Relevant tests include thyroid function tests (fT4 and thyroid-stimulating hormone), insulin tolerance test with measurement of growth hormone and cortisol levels, skull X-ray for evidence of a pituitary tumour and karyotype to exclude Turner's syndrome.

73 Wasted limbs and a distended abdomen. These features are characteristic of intestinal malabsorption syndromes.

74 The association of skeletal fibrous dysplasia, precocious puberty and pigmentation is characteristic of polyostotic fibrous dysplasia (Albright's syndrome).

75 (a) Diabetic gangrene.
(b) Statements (i) and (iv) are true. Adjacent infection with surrounding

cellulitis is common. X-rays often reveal an underlying osteitis. It is always wise to persuade such patients to give up smoking.

76 (a) Children below the third percentile for height warrant further investigation to establish the cause, particularly if there is no family history of short stature. It is important to recognise treatable causes of shortness, e.g., growth hormone deficiency.
(b) Immature facies, plumpness, immature genitalia, particularly a small penis all suggest pituitary failure.

77 (a) The X-ray shows subperiosteal erosions.
(b) Investigation (i) might be helpful. These lesions are characteristic of hyperparathyroidism. Patchy new-bone formation is seen along the phalanges in thyroid acropachy and linear new-bone formation in hypertrophic pulmonary osteoarthropathy and subperiosteal erosions are not seen in these conditions.

78–80 (a) Myxoedema.
(b) (i), (ii) and (iv) are recognised features. Electrocardiographic features of hypothyroidism are non-specific and may mimic ischaemic heart disease or hypertension. They resolve fully with adequate thyroxine medication. It must be remembered that the changes of ischaemic heart disease may co-exist.

81 (a) Monilial angular stomatitis.
(b) Disorders (i), (iii), (iv) and (v) are complicated by this condition. Chronic monilial infection should always raise the possibility of AIDS, particularly in the groups at risk for this infection. Oral contraceptives, corticosteroids and broad-spectrum antibiotic therapy all increase the risk of monilial infection. Anticoagulant therapy does not predispose to moniliasis.

82 (a) Alopecia areata.
(b) Statements (i), (ii) and (iv) are correct. Alopecia areata is associated with any of the organ-specific autoimmune diseases. It responds poorly to therapy, though spontaneous remission is common.

83 (a) The illustration shows dwarfism with very short limbs but a normal trunk length. Thus the upper segment (symphysis pubis to the crown of the head) length is much greater than that of the lower segment. The two segments should be of approximately equal length. The photograph also shows a severe lumbar lordosis.
(b) These features are characteristic of achondroplasia.
(c) Achondroplasia is due to a single autosomal dominant gene although the majority of cases (80%) result from a mutation, since the parents of most affected patients are of average height.

84 (a) Hypothalamic obesity due to the Prader–Willi syndrome.
(b) Statements (i), (ii) and (iii) are true. There is rarely true enlargement of glandular breast tissue and most of the apparent breast swelling is due to fat. The increased appetite is due to derangement of the hypothalamic appetite centre and it is very difficult to limit such patient's food intake. The patients are often mentally retarded. Diabetes mellitus, not diabetes insipidus is a frequent complication. The patients tend to have small hands and feet.

85, 86 (a) Sarcoidosis—the illustrations show a skin lesion and hilar lymphadenopathy.
(b) Sarcoidosis may be associated with hypercalcaemia.

87 (a) The skull X-ray shows an enlarged pituitary fossa. Multiple endocrine neoplasia Type I (MEN I) should be considered.
(b) Statements (iii) and (iv) are correct. MEN I is dominantly inherited

though it can also occur sporadically. Phaeochromocytomas are a feature of MEN II, though there is a rare syndrome in which phaeochromocytomas are associated with acromegaly. MEN I should be considered in all patients with pituitary, parathyroid and pancreatic islet-cell tumours who should be screened for other organ involvement. If a lesion is found in more than one organ on skull X-ray, fasting blood sugar level or serum calcium the same screen should be applied to all first-degree relatives. The tumours are not infrequently malignant hence the term endocrine neoplasia rather than endocrine adenoma.

88 New vessels arising from the disc. Formation of new vessels is the most important of all retinal lesions. They are most serious when they arise on or adjacent to the optic disc or macula. Haemorrhage is frequent and may extend into the vitreous. As it becomes organised it leads to fibrosis and may cause retinal detachment and tearing.

89 Proliferative retinopathy also arising from the disc and mimicking papilloedema.

90 (a) The illustration shows a 45 XO karyotype characteristic of Turner's syndrome.
(b) Statements (i) and (iii) are true. Patients with Turner's syndrome are phenotypically female and characteristically are sexually immature. Clitoral hypertrophy may very rarely be seen in Turner's mosaics with a Y cell line.

91 (a) Graves' disease.
(b) Signs (ii) and (iii) are exhibited. Lid retraction, as indicated by the visibility of sclera between the upper lid and the cornea, is not present. Sclera is visible between the cornea and the lower lid which indicates the presence of exophthalmos. Periorbital swelling is present, particularly above the upper lids. The variety illustrated here is non-specific and can be seen in the presence of any space-occupying orbital lesion. Congestive ophthalmopathy, a term preferred to malignant exophthalmos, is not present. In congestive ophthalmology the lids are infiltrated and often reddened, the conjunctivae are injected, there is chemosis and evidence of active inflammation. So far as can be seen, the ocular axes are parallel and there is no evidence of ophthalmoplegia shown here, though a full range of eye movements would be required to exclude muscle paresis.

92 All of these. Renal hypercalciuria and primary hyperparathyroidism are associated with an increased urinary calcium load. There is moderate hypercalciuria in renal tubular acidosis but this is compounded by increased saturation of calcium phosphate (due to the high urinary pH) and impaired inhibitory activity (due to defective citrate excretion). Cystine stones are opaque since they contain sulphur.

93 (a) Hypospadias, bifid scrotum and testicular atrophy.
(b) These abnormalities are characteristic of Reifenstein's syndrome—a condition limited to males, inherited as an X-linked recessive or as a male-limited autosomal dominant.

94 Cushing's syndrome. Excess circulating glucocorticoid causes growth retardation in children and adolescents. Congenital adrenal hyperplasia causes acceleration of growth although this is followed by early fusion of the epiphyses and thus the final height is reduced.

95 (a) Fine wrinkling of the skin in the circumoral region.
(b) (iii) and (v) may be associated. Fine wrinkling of the skin associated with absence of facial hair is characteristic of hypogonadism in the adult male and

may be due to primary testicular failure or secondary to pituitary failure.

96 (a) Acromegaly with thyroid enlargement.
(b) Statements (i) to (v) are all true. Goitre is common in acromegaly but most patients are euthyroid. Nodular goitres are common and evidence has been produced that the goitre results from a growth-hormone-induced rise in hepatic somatomedin-C production. Thyroid hormone binding protein abnormalities are common and vary with the stage and activity of the disease.

97 (a) Von Recklinghausen's disease (a neuroectodermal disorder). The picture shows the characteristic neurofibromas and the associated irregular and asymmetric café-au-lait pigmentation.
(b) There is an association between the neuroectodermal disorders and phaeochromocytoma.

98 Statements (ii) and (iv) are correct. The screening test of choice is not measurement of the thyroxine but of TSH on the Guthrie spot. Neonatal hypothyroidism due to pituitary disease is very much rarer than that due to primary thyroid disease. Transplacental passage of TSH-receptor blocking antibodies is a rare cause of transient neonatal hypothyroidism affecting particularly women with myxoedema or Hashimoto's disease. The physical signs of neonatal hypothyroidism are non-specific and it is difficult to establish an early diagnosis by clinical means.

99 (a) A nodular goitre.
(b) Statement (iii) is correct. She does not feature eye signs of Graves' disease. Malignancy is rarely associated with a typical nodular goitre. Most long-standing cases of nodular goitre are thought to have arisen as a result of previous iodine deficiency though this is difficult to prove. At this stage, iodine administration would not help the goitre, and in fact might precipitate hyperthyroidism, the so called Jod–Basedow phenomenon. Thyrotrophin-receptor antibodies, the cause of the hyperthyroidism and goitre of Graves' disease are not found in a nodular goitre unless Graves' disease develops in a patient with a pre-existing nodular goitre.

100 (a) Cushing's syndrome.
(b) Obesity (from increased deposition of fat in fat depots), oedema (from increased mineralocorticoid production) and back pain (from osteoporosis) may all be present.

101 (a) The Verner–Morrison syndrome which results from a VIPoma.
(b) Abnormalities (i), (ii), (iv) and (v) accompany this condition. This syndrome is associated with dehydration, hypokalaemia, hypochlorhydria and elevated levels of VIP and PP.

102 The loss of the lamina dura is a characteristic radiological finding of hyperparathyroidism. A raised serum calcium is a characteristic finding in hyperparathyroidism.

103 (a) Rickets.
(b) Disorders (i) and (ii) (directly) and (v) (indirectly). Rickets is caused by vitamin D deficiency (due to dietary deficiency or malabsorption), impaired action (in a range of disorders which includes renal tubular acidosis) or through increased catabolism (which may result from commonly used enzyme-inducing anti-epileptic drugs such as phenytoin).

104 (a) Non-insulin dependent diabetes mellitus associated with gross obesity.
(b) Statements (i), (iii) and (v) are true. Post-mortem studies have shown a 30–50% decrease in B-cell mass. Islet-cell antibodies are not usually found and

if present suggest that the patient may have a slowly developing form of IDDM and will later require insulin.

105 (a) Vitiligo.
(b) Addison's disease only. Vitiligo is commonly associated with organ-specific autoimmune endocrine (and some other autoimmune) disorders.

106 True hermaphroditism is rare and may be associated with a 46XX or a 46XY karyotype or with a 46XX/XY chimaera. The last are true whole-body chimaeras and other cell markers often indicate that the affected individual carries two genetically distinct cell lines.

107 (a) Hirsutism extending up the midline—a male pattern of distribution.
(b) Conditions (i), (ii) and (iii) may be responsible. This may result from an increase in androgens of adrenal or ovarian origin. The latter was the case in this instance, since the patient had the polycystic ovary syndrome.

108 (a) The X-ray shows an osteoclastoma.
(b) Osteoclastomas (giant cell tumours; brown tumours) may be associated with hyperparathyroiditism, and these tumours are frequently indistinguishable, radiologically and histologically, from spontaneous osteoclastomas. (Paget's disease may give rise to an osteosarcoma but this is rare.)

109, 110 (a) The initial scan shows a hypodense lesion compatible with a prolactinoma. The scan taken during pregnancy shows expansion of the tumour with a significant suprasellar extension.
(b) Statements (i), (ii) and (iv) are correct. Prolactinomas often increase in size during pregnancy. The typical symptoms of an expanding pituitary tumour are described. The field defect is characteristically a bitemporal hemianopia, though a homonymous hemianopia can rarely occur depending on the location of the chiasm and the spread of the tumour. All women with pituitary tumours who become pregnant should have monthly field checks. Expansion of a prolactinoma during pregnancy is an indication for bromocriptine therapy for which no teratogenic effects have been demonstrated.

111 (iii) fits the picture. The investigations indicate an increase in adrenal androgen production. There is an increase in ACTH, since cortisol production is impaired, and this causes a secondary increase in adrenal androgen production. The 21-hydroxylase defect characterised by a raised plasma 17α-OH-progesterone is much more common than the 11β-hydroxylase defect and the latter can usually be recognised by the presence of hypertension and elevation of plasma 11- deoxycortisol.

112 (a) A drug-induced goitre should be seriously considered in any patient with asthma since iodine-containing cough medicines are commonly used by asthmatics.
(b) Statements (ii), (iii) and (v) are true. Goitres are much less common in men and iodine deficiency as a cause of goitre in the UK is very rare indeed. Iodides administered for a variety of reasons are one of the commonest goitrogens.

113 Investigations (ii), (iii), (iv) and (v) may be helpful. The probable cause of this degree of growth retardation in the absence of other symptoms is growth hormone deficiency. Circulating growth hormone (GH) levels are low in many fasting normal subjects. It is necessary to demonstrate a failure of GH to rise on stimulation and this is customarily carried out with insulin or arginine in children. A skull X-ray may show an abnormality of the pituitary fossa. Severe hypothyroidism may also lead to growth retardation. A raised thyrotrophin in association with a low thyroxine would indicate primary hypothyroidism.

114 (a) Leucotrichia—which is associated with vitiligo.

(b) Conditions (i), (iii) and (iv) are associated. Leuchotrichia, vitiligo and Turner's syndrome are all associated with organ-specific autoimmune disorders.

115 Statements (ii), (iii), (iv) and (v) are correct. The insulin gene is located on the short arm of chromosome 11.

116 Statements (i), (ii) and (iv) are true. The characteristic karyotype is XXY but occasionally other abnormalities—XY/XXY mosaics, XXYY, XXXY, XXXYY, and XXXXY are seen.

117 Investigation (i) is required. Growth hormone is secreted in a pulsatile manner and also in response to stress. The diagnosis is confirmed by demonstrating that GH levels do not suppress during a glucose tolerance test. Arginine and hypoglycaemia both stimulate the secretion of GH and are used in the investigation of possible GH deficiency. A skull X-ray may show expansion of the pituitary fossa. This is not essential to establish the diagnosis, although if present it would make the diagnosis highly likely.

118 (a) Nelson's syndrome.

(b) (i), (iii) and (iv) are regular features. Patients with Nelson's syndrome have raised and often very high levels of circulating ACTH which leads to the increased melanin deposition in the skin. Normally they have had complete bilateral adrenalectomies and their cortisol levels will depend only on the dose of administered corticosteroid. The expanding corticotroph adenoma often but not invariably causes expansion of the pituitary fossa. Diabetes insipidus is not commonly a feature, unless the tumour is very large and has extended into the suprasellar region.

119 Depression, simple obesity and chronic alcoholism. The majority of patients referred with a possible diagnosis of Cushing's syndrome are simply obese but they may have other clinical features suggesting Cushing's syndrome such as hirsutism or plethora. Depression may cause particular problems, since it is a common feature of Cushing's syndrome, and a patient with endogenous depression may not show a normal circadian rhythm of cortisol secretion. Chronic alcoholism may also mimic the clinical features of Cushing's syndrome. Hypothyroidism and essential hypertension (unless associated with obesity) should not be confused clinically with Cushing's syndrome.

120 (a) Diabetes mellitus.

(b) (i), (iii) and (iv) are shown. There is no evidence of choroidoretinitis or a pre-retinal haemorrhage.

121 These findings are characteristic of anorexia nervosa. Acromegaly is excluded by the suppression of growth hormone levels by glucose. Weight loss and raised growth hormone levels are not features of Cushing's syndrome or premature ovarian failure, and the other physical characteristics of these conditions are not present.

122 Statements (ii), (iii) and (iv) are true. Undescended testes will not descend at puberty without treatment. They must be distinguished from retractile testes which can generally be massaged into the scrotum. There is a considerably enhanced risk of malignancy in undescended testes particularly if they remain in the abdomen. Surgical treatment should be carried out if descent is not induced by hCG (or gonadotrophin-releasing hormone).

123, 124 (a) The X-rays show lytic lesions in the skull and acetabulum, in this context suggestive of eosinophilic granuloma.

(b) Statements (i) to (v) are all true. Eosinophilic granuloma can occur in adults as well as in children. It is usually a benign condition. It may present with a spontaneous pneumothorax. Lung infiltration may occur and hypothalamic involvement commonly causes diabetes insipidus.

125 (a) Clitoral hypertrophy.
(b) Features (i), (ii) and (iii) are associated. Clitoral hypertrophy results from excess circulating androgen and may be seen in congenital adrenal hyperplasia, masculinising tumours, Cushing's syndrome, due to administration of masculinising drugs or secondary to carcinomas of the kidney or ovary. It may, therefore, be associated with hirsutism or shortness of stature since excess circulating androgen will lead to accelerated skeletal development and early epiphyseal closure. Hypertension may be associated with clitoral hypertrophy in Cushing's syndrome and in some forms of congenital adrenal hyperplasia (particularly 11ß-hydroxylase deficiency).

126, 127 (a) Two large flat-topped subhyaloid haemorrhages are shown. These are seen in diabetes mellitus and after a subarachnoid haemorrhage.
(b) Changes (i), (ii), (iii) and (v) are shown. The subhyaloid haemorrhages are pre-retinal, i.e. in front of the retinal vessels which can be demonstrated by giving intravascular fluorescein.

128 Statements (ii) and (iv) are true. A medial strabismus would be expected in the presence of a sixth nerve palsy. She has clear evidence of a cataract and the lateral concomitant strabismus is the result of a myopic amblyopic left eye of long-standing. Apart from prominence of the left eye there are no other ocular features of Graves' disease. Seen beyond the cataract are typical features of a myopic fundus. The condition is irreversible and no treatment would help the prominence of the eye or improve the visual acuity.

129, 130 (a) **129** shows active acromegaly and **130** an apparently normal woman. Explanation (i) is that **130** is a result of treatment and suggests cured acromegaly. Explanation (ii) would be that **130** is the patient before the onset of acromegaly.
(b) Criteria (i), (ii) and (iii) are true. There is usually a rapid and marked reduction in size of the hands and feet, and in soft-tissue swelling, causing obvious improvement in facial appearance. Patients with cured acromegaly show suppression of GH levels to <1.0 mU/l, older criteria of <10 or <5 mU/l are outmoded. Patients with acromegaly often show a GH response to TRH and loss of this response is a feature of cure. Similarly a proportion of acromegalics show a GH response to GnRH and this is lost when the disease is cured.

131 (a) Menopausal flush.
(b) Statements (i), (iii) and (v) are true. The flushes often commence before the menopause and may continue up to a decade afterwards. Circulating oestrogen levels are lowered and serum FSH elevated. They respond promptly to oestrogen medication.

132, 133 (a) **132** shows an empty pituitary fossa and a centrally placed stalk; **133** is a CT scan with contrast medium filling the fossa, confirming the presence of the 'empty fossa syndrome'.
(b) Statements (i) to (vi) are all correct. The pituitary fossa is often enlarged. The 'empty fossa syndrome' may be the late result of infarction of a pituitary tumour but this is not common. Benign intracranial hypertension may lead to the syndrome. Pituitary hormone levels are usually normal, though a minor elevation of prolactin may be seen. Congenital deficiency of the diaphragm sellae is the commonest cause of the syndrome for which no treatment is required.

134 (a) The diabetic hand syndrome.
(b) Statements (i), (ii), (iii) and (v) are true. The characteristic features of the diabetic hand syndrome are a waxy skin and joint contractures with limited movement of the joints. It may be associated with Dupuytren's contractures.

135 Conditions (ii) and (v) may be associated. There is a rare association between hypothyroidism and precocious puberty which may result from secondary disturbance of hypothalamic function. Tumours in the pineal region probably cause precocious puberty by pressure on the hypothalamus.

136 (a) Paget's disease of bone.
(b) Statement (ii) is true. The bone lesions may also be seen in the pelvis, vertebral column and skull. Paget's disease is most frequent in the USA, Western Europe and Australasia. The majority of patients with Paget's disease are asymptomatic although bone pain may occur in a minority of patients.

137 (a) Pigmentation of the buccal cavity, suggesting the possibility of Addison's disease.
(b) Plasma cortisol and its response to depot ACTH 8 and 24 hours after the dose, which should exceed 700 nmol/l. Plasma ACTH is raised.

138 (a) Endemic goitre related to iodine deficiency.
(b) Statements (i), (ii), (iii) and (iv) are correct. Iodine deficiency is the major factor leading to endemic goitre, but in certain areas ingestion of goitrogens, e.g., thiocyanate from cassava, may contribute to the thyroid abnormality. Most adults with endemic goitre are clinically euthyroid though some exhibit biochemical features of hypothyroidism. Endemic cretinism is a feature of areas of severe iodine deficiency and can be prevented by the administration of iodised oil either orally or intramuscularly to women at risk of pregnancy or in early pregnancy.

139 (a) Reduced bone density, severe kyphosis, diminished vertebral height and a crush fracture. These changes are characteristic of osteoporosis.
(b) Severe osteoporosis may result from accelerated bone loss due to premature ovarian failure or from increased catabolism due to Cushing's syndrome.

140 (a) The features described are characteristic of Marfan's syndrome in which tallness of stature is associated with a variety of somatic abnormalities.
(b) (ii), (iii) and (iv) may be present. Marfan's syndrome is characterised by laxity of the ligaments and structural abnormalities of collagen which lead to a range of somatic manifestations.

141 (a) Pseudo gout—the patient is most likely to suffer from progressive degenerative joint disease indistinguishable clinically from osteoarthrosis. An acute arthritis (crystal synovitis) resulting from the precipitation of crystals of calcium pyrophosphate, hydroxyapatite and orthophosphate is less common.
(b) Disorders (ii), (iii) and (iv)—all three of these conditions can lead to the deposition of calcium salts in the joints. Hyperuricaemia gives rise to a crystal synovitis (gout) but urate is not radio-opaque.

142 (a) Gynaecomastia of puberty.
(b) Statements (i), (iii) and (v) are true. It is a very common manifestation of normal puberty and is quite often tender. It usually remits spontaneously but often causes significant embarrassment and psychological upset. If it persists, surgical removal of breast tissue may be considered.

143 Nelson's syndrome results from greatly increased ACTH levels (ACTH is the melanotrophic hormone) following bilateral adrenalectomy for hypothalamic–pituitary driven Cushing's syndrome (Cushing's disease). It occurs despite adequate replacement therapy. Muscle weakness may occur and skin fragility due to the previous cortisol excess may persist for many years.

144 Ullrich–Turner syndrome (also known as 'male' Turner's or Noonan's syndrome) has these features and the patients may also exhibit the other somatic features of Turner's syndrome in the female.

145 Congenital adrenal hyperplasia. The findings indicate an increase in androgen production due to an inherited abnormality of steroid biosynthesis. Similar findings on investigation would be found in a patient with an arrhenoblastoma but such a tumour would not be found before puberty and thus the patient would have secondary and not primary amenorrhoea.

146 (a) The picture shows the dry tongue of a dehydrated diabetic with ketoacidosis.
(b) Complications (i), (ii) and (iii) are seen. In the volume-depleted dehydrated diabetic with ketoacidosis, skin turgor is reduced and there is hypotension, tachycardia and a low-volume pulse. There is often evidence of a precipitating infection. Papilloedema and acute neuropathy are not recognised features of ketoacidosis.

147 (a) Facial hirsutism.
(b) (ii), (iii) and (iv) may be responsible. Hirsutism is a recognised complication of prolonged phenytoin therapy. The mechanism is unknown. Hirsutism may also accompany the administration of pharmacological doses of those glucocorticoids which have some androgenic action. It is seen infrequently in patients treated with prednisolone.

148 (a) Onycholysis.
(b) Statements (i), (ii) and (v) are true. Onycholysis is a known association of hyperthyroidism. Onycholysis also occurs in psoriasis where pitting of the nails is an additional sign. Iron deficiency does not contribute to onycholysis, though it is a known cause of koilonychia. Onycholysis is not specifically related to localised myxoedema. No local treatment of the nails is effective or required.

149 Hypothyroidism. All of these endocrine conditions may lead to growth retardation, but growth failure of this severity in the absence of other symptoms is unlikely to be due to adrenal failure, hypoparathyroidism or diabetes mellitus. The diagnosis can be confirmed by finding low circulating thyroid hormone levels and, if of thyroid origin, a raised thyrotrophin (TSH).

150 (a) Osteoporosis.
(b) (iv) and (v) may cause this abnormality. Hypercortisolism from any cause leads to osteoporosis due to increased protein catabolism.

151, 152 (a) Multiple endocrine neoplasia (MEN) Type IIb (Sipple's syndrome).
(b) (i), (ii), (iii) and (iv) are features. Mucosal neuromas are seen on the lips, eyelids and tongue. A proximal myopathy may be associated. 'C cell' hyperplasia or neoplasia with elevation of calcitonin is a marker of the disease. Phaeochromocytomas and adrenal medullary hyperplasia are usually bilateral. Islet-cell adenomas are part of MEN I and are not associated with MEN II.

153 These clinical and radiological features are characteristic of multiple epiphyseal dysplasia (Fairbank's syndrome). This is probably a heterogeneous group of disorders inherited as an autosomal dominant, although an autosomal recessive variety has also been described. The epiphyseal abnormalities predispose to degenerative joint disease. Osteogenesis imperfecta is associated with a history of multiple fractures and the epiphyseal abnormalities are not present. Rickets is associated with widening and cupping of the epiphyseal plates. Specific epiphyseal abnormalities are not seen in hypoparathyroidism.

154 (a) There is enlargement of the pituitary fossa, and the pattern of enlargement, with a 'square-shaped' fossa, is typical of acromegaly.
(b) Statements (i), (ii) and (iii) are correct. Acromegaly often develops insidiously and may be asymptomatic. Compression of the median nerve at the wrist, by increased bone and soft-tissue growth in the region of the carpal tunnel, frequently results in acroparaesthesiae. Hypertension is common in acromegaly though the underlying mechanism is poorly understood. To exclude acromegaly, GH levels should be suppressed to < 1 mU/l during a standard glucose tolerance test. The pituitary fossa is enlarged in about 90% of acromegalics, the more severe the acromegaly and the higher the GH levels, the larger the fossa but a normal fossa does not exclude acromegaly.

155 (a) Looser's zone (a partial fracture surrounded by a denser zone of callus). The lesion is characteristic of osteomalacia.
(b) Muscle weakness, particularly affecting the pelvic girdle and thigh muscles, is a common presenting symptom of osteomalacia. Bone tenderness may occur in severe disease.

156 These clinical findings, which are also associated with small hands and feet, and mental retardation, are characteristic of the Prader–Willi syndrome.

157 (a) The diabetes of acromegaly is not usually complicated by ketoacidosis.
(b) All of the conditions listed, apart from a non-secretory pituitary adenoma, may be complicated by diabetes mellitus.

158 (a) Hypoparathyroidism—intracranial and particularly basal ganglia calcification is seen in about one-third of patients.
(b) (i), (ii) and (iii) may be associated. Epilepsy is common and is resistant to anti-convulsant drugs alone, but fits disappear when the hypocalcaemia is treated. Papilloedema occurs, although its cause is not well understood. The clinical features of basal ganglia disturbances may occur, although the pattern of these often does not match the distribution of the calcification.

159 (a) Statement (ii) is correct. The right ocular axis is displaced downwards and this suggests an orbital space-occupying lesion rather than ophthalmic Graves' disease. He lacks lid retraction and periorobital swelling which you would expect to see in Graves' disease.
(b) X-ray of the orbit. In this case an X-ray of the orbit revealed a break in the continuity of the bone which was due to a mucocele of the right frontal sinus, impinging on the orbit. A CT scan would clearly demonstrate the presence of the mucocele. Operative intervention was required to demonstrate the mucocele and drain it, and to exclude local malignancy.

160 (a) Purple striae.
(b) Cushing's syndrome.
(c) Striae are commonly seen in obese patients, and although these are usually white or pink in colour, they may be purple and differentiation on purely clinical grounds may be difficult.
(d) Thinning and stretching of the skin due to protein loss from increased protein catabolism.
(e) No. Purple striae may be seen in non-parous women and men with Cushing's syndrome and occasionally in men with obesity.

161 (a) Primary hypothyroidism (myxoedema).
(b) Statements (i) to (v) are all true. Depressive symptoms are common in

hypothyroidism. Ptosis is a known feature and remits with thyroxine therapy. Myasthenia gravis is a known association of autoimmune thyroid disease and in the presence of ptosis myasthenia should be excluded by a tensilon test. Ptosis can also occur as a rare manifestation of Graves' ophthalmopathy, and again myasthenia gravis must be excluded. Body cavity effusions are not uncommon in hypothyroidism and include pericardial effusion, ascites, uveal effusion, pleural effusion and hydroceles. Most patients with spontaneous hypothyroidism in the UK are found to be suffering from autoimmune thyroid disease and they commonly show circulating anti-thyroid peroxidase antibodies, previously referred to as anti-microsomal antibodies.

162 Statements (ii), (iv) and (v) are true. These features are characteristic of gonadal dysgenesis associated with an XX karyotype. The syndrome may also be seen with an XY karyotype and such patients are also phenotypically female. The risk of malignancy in the dysgenetic male gonad is even greater than in the female.

163 (a) A recurrent left upper pole thyroid nodule, regrown from residual thyroid tissue left at the time of the previous operation.
(b) Investigations (i) to (v) would all be helpful. TRAb levels would indicate whether her Graves' disease remained active; ultrasound whether the nodule was cystic, solid, or calcified; and ^{123}I scan whether the nodule was functional. Calcium and phosphate levels are always worth checking after a previous thyroidectomy, to exclude hypoparathyroidism. A fine-needle biopsy would be useful to exclude a thyroid carcinoma or coincidental malignancy.

164 (a) Tetany—the picture shows the typical contraction producing the *main d'accoucheur*.
(b) Hypocalcaemia and hypomagnesaemia cause neural hyperexcitability leading directly to tetany. Hypokalaemia does so indirectly by causing an alkalosis.

165 There are a number of causes of low birth weight shortness of stature. These include placental insufficiency, intrauterine infections and many autosomal chromosomal anomalies. In monozygotic twins, the last two possibilities would have affected both of the pair. The direct cause was severe placental insufficiency affecting one twin only.

166 (a) A thyroglossal cyst (alternative correct answer, an ectopic thyroid).
(b) Statements (i), (iii) and (iv) are true. Thyroid function is variably impaired in patients with a thyroglossal cyst, depending on whether they have additional normal functioning thyroid tissue. Because of long-standing elevated thyroid-stimulating hormone levels there is an increased risk of malignancy. The serum calcitonin level remains normal.

167 (a) Female breast showing pigmentation of the nipple.
(b) This could be of racial origin. Pregnancy and stilboestrol therapy lead to pigmentation of the nipples. The raised ACTH levels seen in untreated Addison's disease cause generalised pigmentation, including darkening of the nipples.

168 (a) Graves' disease, described by Parry in 1825, Graves in 1835 and von Basedow in 1840. She illustrates bilateral lid retraction, periorbital swelling, and a moderate goitre.
(b) Amiodarone, the anti-arrhythmic drug, can cause hyperthyroidism because of its high iodine content. Post-partum thyroiditis is probably the commonest cause of hyperthyroidism, affecting about 10% of women 3 months after delivery. The hyperthyroidism is rarely symptomatic and is revealed by transient abnormalities of the thyroid function tests. Bronchogenic carcinoma

producing an ectopic thyroid-stimulating hormone (TSH) syndrome has not been definitively described. Choriocarcinoma, where circulating levels of human chorionic gonadotrophin (hCG) are very high, may cause hyperthyroidism because of interaction of the hCG with the TSH receptor on the thyroid follicular cells. De Quervain's viral thyroiditis is a rare cause of a destructive thyroiditis with hyperthyroidism in the earlier stages of the disease.

169, 170 (a) Thyroid acropachy.
(b) Statements (ii), (iii) and (v) are correct. The nail changes shown are typical of the thyroid acropachy of Graves' disease. Most patients with thyroid acropachy also show evidence of localised myxoedema and in both conditions there are high levels of circulating thyrotrophin receptor antibodies. Thyroid acropachy rarely remits even with effective treatment. X-ray of the hands can be used to differentiate thyroid acropachy from hypertrophic pulmonary osteoarthropathy. In the former, subperiosteal new-bone formation is patchy, resembling soap bubbles on the surface of the bone, whereas in the latter the sub-periosteal new bone has a linear distribution.

171 (a) Polyostotic fibrous dysplasia (Albright's syndrome).
(b) All of these have been reported to be associated with polyostotic fibrous dysplasia. It is generally assumed that the precocious puberty results from compression of the hypothalamus due to deformity of the bones at the base of the skull. The mechanism responsible for these abnormalities is still not understood.

172 Conditions (i) and (iii)—the bone changes in these are associated with precocious puberty leading to accelerated skeletal maturity and premature epiphyseal closure. In pinealomas, these changes are almost certainly due to pressure on the hypothalamus with secondary endocrine disturbance.

173 (a) An enlarged pituitary fossa. You should consider the probability that she has an ectopic thyroid, with mild long-standing thyroid failure, causing feedback hyperplasia of the pituitary thyrotroph cells.
(b) (i), (iii), (iv) are recognised features. Thyrotroph hyperplasia may progress to adenoma formation and the enlarged pituitary may compress the optic chiasm. The serum TSH level is usually grossly elevated at > 100 mU/l but responds, as does the pituitary hyperplasia, to adequate thyroxine replacement. Shortness of stature may result from the long-standing thyroid failure. There is no increased prevalence of thyroid antibodies in patients with an ectopic thyroid.

174 (a) Acromegaly.
(b) Statements (ii), (iii), (iv) and (v) are true. Acromegaly is usually due to a somatotroph adenoma of the pituitary; rarely acromegaly may result from ectopic production of GRF by a tumour, commonly a pancreatic neoplasm. Macroglossia is common in acromegaly. Increased skin thickness is a cardinal physical sign of acromegaly. Galactorrhoea is common in acromegaly, due either to the lactogenic action of growth hormone and/or concomitant overproduction of prolactin.

175, 176 Statements (i), (iii), (iv) and (v) are correct. Children with neonatal hyperthyroidism usually have detectable thyroid enlargement. The mother became hypothyroid after radioiodine therapy, and her thyroid has probably shrunk to an undetectable size. Urgent tests are required to confirm the diagnosis, meanwhile treatment with iodine and carbimazole should be initiated at once. Mothers of such children usually have eye signs of Graves' disease, localised myxoedema and high circulating levels of TRAb. Neonatal hyperthyroidism results from transplacental passage of TRAb and remits with a half life of IgG (about 20–30 days).

177 (a) Gigantism with some features of acromegaly and hypopituitarism.
(b) Excessive tallness and coarse features, bilateral gynaecomastia, large hands and feet, and lack of sexual development. Lateral skull X-ray, to show the enlarged pituitary fossa; and glucose tolerance test with measurement of growth hormone (GH) levels, to establish raised basal levels and lack of suppression of GH to < 1.0 mU/l.

178 (a) The X-ray shows cardiac enlargement, and is of a female as indicated by the breast shadows.
(b) Hypertension occurs more frequently in acromegaly than the general population, although the mechanism is not understood. Ischaemic heart disease is common in acromegalics with diabetes mellitus. Acromegalic cardiomyopathy is a known and dangerous complication of long-standing acromegaly. It can occasionally be ameliorated by lowering the growth hormone levels substantially by adenomectomy or by drug therapy with bromocriptine or somatostatin analogues. Pericardial effusion and amyloidosis are not associated with acromegaly.

179 (a) Conns' syndrome.
(b) Hypertension and severe muscle weakness are characteristic of the syndrome, resulting from sodium retention and potassium depletion respectively, due to mineralocorticoid excess. Tetany is common due to hypokalaemic alkalosis. Oedema is rare in Conn's syndrome.

180 (a) Cushing's syndrome.
(b) Amenorrhoea (due to increased androgen secretion) is an almost invariable feature in Cushing's syndrome, and depression is also common. Bronchospasm and diarrhoea are not primary clinical features of Cushing's syndrome, but the ectopic ACTH syndrome may be caused by a carcinoid tumour which may also give rise to these symptoms.

181 (a) Xanthelasma.
(b) Statements (i), (iii), (iv) and (v) are true. Xanthelasma is more often seen in hypothyroidism, where the serum cholesterol level is frequently raised.

182 (a) Juvenile hypothyroidism is easily overlooked and is always accompanied by a reduced rate of growth.
(b) Prolactin levels are often raised, leading to galactorrhoea. Sexual precocity may be seen in either sex and serum follicle-stimulating hormone levels are invariably raised. Pigmentation of the skin and nephrocalcinosis are rare but ill-understood manifestations of juvenile hypothyroidism.

183, 184 (a) The glucagonoma syndrome.
(b) Statements (i) and (iii) are true. Glossitis, often severe, is common and the rash can be induced by administration of glucagon, but is not helped by magnesium. The associated diabetes is usually mild and not accompanied by ketoacidosis.

185–187 (a) These pictures show achilles tendon xanthomas and typical eruptive xanthomas, often seen over the elbows and buttocks.
(b) Statements (i) and (iv) are true. Cholesterol, LDL–cholesterol and triglyceride levels are raised in diabetes. Tendon xanthomas normally resolve with good control of the diabetes.

188 Diagnoses (i) and (v) fit. These results will only be found in women given androgens if the natural hormone is given—testosterone levels will be suppressed if a synthetic compound has been administered. Raised levels of testosterone and reduced levels of SHBG are found in congenital adrenal hyperplasia and virilising adrenal adenomas but the urinary 17-oxogenic and oxosteroid levels will also be raised.

189 Testicular feminisation (a highly distinctive inherited disorder in genotypic males), in which there is tissue resistance to androgens and thus wolffian duct structures are poorly developed. Feminisation probably results from increased oestrogen levels (for a male) which are driven by the relatively high gonadotrophins, because of the insensitivity of the normal feedback mechanism to androgens.

190 (a) Fine wrinkling of the skin, which occurs in gonadal and growth hormone (GH) deficiency. It also occurs in the elderly, so the age of the patient must be borne in mind.
(b) Features (i), (ii), (iii) and (iv) might confirm this. Fine wrinkling of the skin is a feature of gonadal deficiency. Loss of pubic hair is common in hypogonadism but also occurs in the elderly, in women with adrenal insufficiency, and in occasional normal individuals. Low free testosterone levels are characteristic of hypogonadism and low LH and FSH levels are typical of pituitary hypogonadism.

191 (a) An enlarged pituitary fossa with backward displacement of the posterior clinoids and calcification in the fossa, suggesting a suprasellar space-occupying lesion such as a craniopharyngioma.
(b) All of the conditions listed may be associated with a craniopharyngioma due to pressure on particular hypothalamic structures. Damage to the mamillary bodies may cause impairment of short-term memory.

192 Soto's syndrome (cerebral gigantism). The other syndromes are all associated with abnormal tallness of stature, but the other clinical features are not present (apart from a high arched palate, which is also found in Marfan's syndrome).

193 Investigations (i), (iii) and (iv) might help in identification. The illustration shows melanosis. The increased melanin deposition may be associated with: bronchial carcinoma; melanoma (and some other malignant tumours); Addison's disease (although this depth of pigmentation would be very rare); Nelson's syndrome (post-adrenalectomy syndrome); and haemochromatosis (in which there is increased deposition of melanin as well as iron containing pigments). This patient had a melanoma removed from her leg 20 years previously.

194 (a) Increased carrying angle at the elbow (cubitus valgus)—an abnormality which is characteristic of Turner's syndrome.
(b) Features (i), (ii) and (iii)—Turner's syndrome may be associated with a wide range of somatic abnormalities.

195 (a) Expansion of the skull bones, loss of cortico-medullary definition and a coarse trabecular pattern. These changes are due to Paget's disease.
(b) The predominant biochemical feature of Paget's disease is a raised serum alkaline phosphatase.

196 (a) Lipaemia retinalis.
(b) Statements (ii) and (iv) are true. Endogenous insulin secretion can be estimated by measuring circulating C-peptide. Patients presenting with untreated IDDM are often ketotic. IDDM is associated with the HLA antigens DR3 and DR4.

197 (a) Chronic fungal infection—probably candidiasis.
(b) Conditions (ii) and (iv)—hyperglycaemic patients are prone to a wide range of infections including mucocutaneous candidiasis, and prolonged hypocalcaemia from any cause predisposes to candidal infection.

198 (a) Papilloedema.
(b) Statements (ii), (iv) and (v) are correct. Papilloedema is rare in patients with pituitary tumours, and would always indicate the presence of a suprasellar extension. Bitemporal hemianopia, though typical of a suprasellar extension is not invariably present and there may not be any visual defect. Papilloedema not infrequently progresses to optic atrophy, despite decompression of the chiasm.

199 (a) Osteogenesis imperfecta.
(b) Statements (i), (ii), (iv) and (v) are true. Osteogenesis imperfecta is generally inherited as an autosomal dominant—Types I and IV (most cases resulting from a mutation). Types II and III, which constitute a minority of cases, show an autosomal recessive pattern of inheritance. Deafness may occur since there is an association with osteosclerosis. Patients may also have hypoplastic teeth.

200 Statements (ii) and (iv) are true. Approximately 10% of lesions are found outside the adrenal. Paroxysmal hypertension is characteristic, although the tumours may also cause a sustained rise in blood pressure. Approximately 10% of tumours are malignant, phaeochromocytoma accounts for only 0.1–0.5% of cases of hypertension and phentolamine will lower the blood pressure in a proportion of cases of essential hypertension.

201–203 (a) Laser burns to the retina.
(b) Statements (i), (ii) and (iii) are correct. It can be used in all varieties of diabetes with appropriate retinopathy.

204 Statements (i) and (iv) are correct. Pigmentation in Cushing's syndrome results from an increase in ACTH production. ACTH is suppressed in adrenal adenoma.

205 (a) Two Barr bodies (condensed chromatin) are seen on the nuclear membrane.
(b) Condition (iii) (occasionally) and (iv). The number of Barr bodies is one less than the number of X chromosomes. Thus there is one in the buccal smear of the normal female and they are absent in the normal male. Two Barr bodies are only seen rarely in patients with Klinefelter's syndrome, since they more commonly have an XXY chromosome constitution and only rarely XXXY.

206 (a) The child shows the characteristic appearance of kwashiorkor which results from severe protein/calorie malnutrition.
(b) Hypoalbuminaemia—serum albumin levels are substantially reduced in kwashiorkor, contributing to the hypoproteinaemic oedema and ascites. The blood urea and cholesterol levels are also low in Kwashiorkor.

207 (a) Adrenocortical carcinoma.
(b) Statements (ii), (iii), (iv) and (vi) are true. The gynaecomastia is likely to be due to oestrogen secretion by the tumour and such lesions tend to secrete androgens, oestrogens and corticosteroids as well as biologically inactive metabolites. The urinary 17-oxosteroid excretion is usually elevated. Prognosis is poor and 5-year survival unlikely.

208 (a) A marked increase in bone density—osteosclerosis.
(b) The most common cause of osteosclerosis is secondary hyper-

parathyroidism due to chronic renal failure. Primary hyperparathyroidism is only rarely associated with osteosclerosis.

209 (a) Absent axillary hair which, if associated with absent or scanty pubic hair in a woman in the reproductive phase of life, is likely to have a pathological origin.
(b) Conditions (i), (iii) and (v) may be responsible, Absent axillary and pubic hair may be seen in conditions in which there is a failure of gonadotrophin production (pituitary failure), androgen deficiency (Addison's disease) or a failure in sexual maturation (Turner's syndrome).

210, 211 (a) McCune–Albright syndrome of polyostotic fibrous dysplasia.
(b) Precocious puberty, acromegaly, hyperthyroidism and Cushing's syndrome.

212 All of these. Any disorder affecting a major organ system or chronic infection may lead to serious growth retardation. This child suffered emotional deprivation, an important cause of growth failure, leading to disturbance of hypothalamic function and, frequently, abnormal responses of growth hormone and ACTH to appropriate stimuli. These changes are reversible if the child's emotional environment is improved.

213 (a) A trophic ulcer.
(b) These are all features of chronic diabetic neuropathy. Sensory nerve involvement is generally distal in distribution and may lead to trophic ulceration. A Charcot joint, a neuropathic arthropathy, can complicate a sensory neuropathy. Motor-nerve involvement causes muscle weakness and wasting, generally proximal in distribution. A mixed peripheral neuropathy, mononeuritis multiplex, can occur. Autonomic neuropathy can cause pupillary changes (Argyll–Robertson pupils), dependent oedema, reduced sweating and bowel, bladder and sphincter disturbance.

214 The association of these clinical features with shortness of stature (illustrated) indicate that the cause is likely to be of hypothalamic-pituitary origin. These endocrine features with blindess due to pressure on the optic pathways suggest the presence of a craniopharyngioma. Patients with Klinefelter's syndrome are generally tall and have gynaecomastia. Patients with the XYY syndrome are often tall, have normal secondary sexual characteristics and are only occasionally hypogonadal. Patients with Ullrich–Turner syndrome are short and do not undergo pubertal changes but they do not suffer from blindness and have the somatic characteristics of the syndrome (i.e., those or Turner's syndrome in the female).

215 (a) Juvenile Graves' disease.
(b) Statements (ii), (iii), (iv) and (v) are true. It is much rarer in children than in adults. It has a strong tendency to relapse and continuous antithyroid drug therapy is often required until thyroidectomy is performed after full pubertal development. A family history of thyroid or other organ-specific autoimmune disease is common. Most patients with Graves' disease have circulating TPO antibodies. It is commonly associated with increased linear growth and in the very young with premature fusion of the skull sutures.

Index

Numbers refer to the number shared by the illustration, question and answer.